DATE DUE

AUG 0 3 2010			

Governors State University
Library Hours:
Monday thru Thursday 8:00 to 10:30
Friday 8:00 to 5:00
Saturday 8:30 to 5:00
Sunday 1:00 to 5:00 (Fall
and Winter Trimester Only)

Kept 12/2013

HEALTH RESEARCH METHODS: A TABULAR PRESENTATION

HEALTH RESEARCH METHODS: A TABULAR PRESENTATION

STEPHEN BUETOW

Nova Biomedical Books
New York

NOTICE TO THE READER

The Publisher has taken reasonable care in the preparation of this book, but makes no expressed or implied warranty of any kind and assumes no responsibility for any errors or omissions. No liability is assumed for incidental or consequential damages in connection with or arising out of information contained in this book. The Publisher shall not be liable for any special, consequential, or exemplary damages resulting, in whole or in part, from the readers' use of, or reliance upon, this material.

Independent verification should be sought for any data, advice or recommendations contained in this book. In addition, no responsibility is assumed by the publisher for any injury and/or damage to persons or property arising from any methods, products, instructions, ideas or otherwise contained in this publication.

This publication is designed to provide accurate and authoritative information with regard to the subject matter covered herein. It is sold with the clear understanding that the Publisher is not engaged in rendering legal or any other professional services. If legal or any other expert assistance is required, the services of a competent person should be sought. FROM A DECLARATION OF PARTICIPANTS JOINTLY ADOPTED BY A COMMITTEE OF THE AMERICAN BAR ASSOCIATION AND A COMMITTEE OF PUBLISHERS.

LIBRARY OF CONGRESS CATALOGING-IN-PUBLICATION DATA
Buetow, Stephen.
 Health research methods : a tabular presentation / Stephen Buetow.
     p. ; cm.
 Includes bibliographical references.
 ISBN-13: 978-1-60021-887-3 (hardcover)
 ISBN-10: 1-60021-887-3 (hardcover)
 1. Health--Research--Methodology. I. Title.
 [DNLM: 1. Biomedical Research--methods--Handbooks. 2. Research Design--Handbooks. W 49 B928h 2007]
 R850.B777 2007
 610.72--dc22

                        2007025739

Published by Nova Science Publishers, Inc. ✦ *New York*

DEDICATION

This book is dedicated to my wife:

Esther Buetow (née Zeland)

CONTENTS

ACKNOWLEDGEMENTS

Numerous groups and individuals have supported me in writing this book. ProCare Health Limited, New Zealand's largest primary care provider network, is thanked for its salary support of my University of Auckland position until the end of 2006. The University of Auckland subsequently took over the permanent funding of this position in its Department of General Practice and Primary Care, School of Population Health, and I greatly appreciate its continuing investment in me.

Individual chapters of this book have benefited from feedback kindly provided by colleagues in the School of Population Health: Associate-Professor Peter Adams, Professor Bruce Arroll, Associate-Professor Timothy Kenealy, Associate-Professor Ngaire Kerse, Mrs. Elizabeth Robinson, Associate-Professor Robert Scragg and Professor David Thomas. The book has also profited from my teaching of a postgraduate health research methods course with School of Nursing Associate-Professors, Robyn Dixon and Jill Bennett, during 2006 and 2007 respectively. The many students that I have had the privilege to teach have further enriched my work. Mrs Elizabeth Kiata provide invaluable assistance with formatting the tables.

All errors by commission or omission in this book are, nevertheless, my responsibility alone.

PREFACE

This book is for busy people who need quick access to robust and easily digestable information on a comprehensive range of health research methods. Such information is needed, first, by those of us who are critical consumers of health research. This book can help us to retrieve, evaluate and use the exponentially increasing volume of new and intricate research evidence to enhance our knowledge base and inform our decision-making, for example in health policy and clinical practice. The book has also been written for people who need research skills for the additional purposes of designing and producing health research and promoting its uptake in practice.

Two approaches are commonly used to manage the use and production of the burgeoning quantity of health research: the literature review and evidence synthesis. These approaches help us to stay abreast of the growth of research and surf the 'knowledge wave' as modern technology transfer puts more wind in our research sails and closes the information distances between us.

However, both approaches have major limitations. They tend to take a narrow focus and to report the use of research methods as a means rather than an end. Designed to be read in full, the literature review and evidence synthesis encourage readers to understand and critically appraise large of amounts of text whose summarized content is dispersed and sequential. But, people cannot quickly and easily process text with these qualities. Although approaches to evidence synthesis offer the potential to aggregate and reconceptualize the findings of individual studies, controversy continues to surround their use to synthesize qualitative and quantitative research.

This book offers a way forward. Intrinsic to literature reviews and evidence synthesis, yet associated more generally with the need to help relieve the cognitive burden of using the maximum information available, is the tendency 'to reduce complex information into selective and simplified gestalts or easily understood configurations' (p. 10) [1]. This process of reduction includes categorization, and underpins the use of tables, graphs, diagrams and maps. Underlying the need for, and organization of, this book is my belief that such summary displays have been underused.

Although extended text will remain the principal medium for communicating detail, there is scope to expand usage of the tabular format to synthesize research and aid learning. This book, therefore, makes increased use of the tabular format. For all those wanting to engage in the critical use or production of health research, including students and teachers of research methods, it decreases the work burden by using tables to summarize essential details and minimize the need to digest large blocks of extended text. Whereas other research methods texts average perhaps 80-90% text and 10-20% tables and other formats, this book does the opposite: at least 80% of the book comprises summary tables (and figures); 20% is text linking the individual tables and chapters.

Drawing on my background as an experienced health researcher, the tables aim to tell readers concisely, yet accurately, what they are most likely to need to know without having to look hard to find it. The tables have also been constructed to be as clear, precise and direct as the tabular format allows. Of course there are costs. The need for concision limits the opportunity to elaborate or explain issues fully. Therefore, although key concepts are defined when first introduced, readers may find it easiest to understand and make optimal use of the tables if they come to this book with at least some basic understanding of research methods or are using the book to support their companion learning in a research methods class. Readers wishing to pursue individual issues in more detail are directed to other, specialized texts referenced at the end of each chapter. The book is based on materials that have formed the foundation of the postgraduate course on health research methods run jointly by the Department of General Practice and Primary Health Care, and the School of Nursing, at the University of Auckland in New Zealand. However, the methodologies and methods covered in the book have relevance beyond health care and are generally applicable to the social sciences.

The book has eight chapters. The first chapter introduces the concept of research and helps readers to situate their own and others' research within basic belief systems. It informs awareness of, and enables reflection on, how different people see the world differently and how their perceptions underpin variation in research questions, choice of methodologies, and the interpretation and implementation of results. Readers are assisted to develop self-awareness of their own beliefs guiding research, and introduced to deductive and inductive routes to explanation. Quantitative and qualitative investigations, as independent and mixed methods, are suggested to offer useful vehicles for traveling along these routes and are detailed in subsequent chapters.

The second chapter suggests how to formulate a good research question and set aims, objectives or hypotheses. It equips readers with a basic vocabulary sufficient to read and plan quantitative health research. In this context the chapter describes the main study designs and demonstrates how to calculate and interpret summary measures of frequency and effect. The chapter concludes by introducing the statistical concepts of p values and confidence intervals.

This provides an entry point to the discussion of literature reviews. Chapter 3 discusses types and sources of literature. It explains the need for literature reviews and summarizes different types of literature review before outlining a stepwise approach to conducting the systematic review. Approaches to evidence synthesis are compared and focus is given to the process of producing respectively a meta-analysis and meta-ethnography. Lastly, the chapter suggests how to critique a systematic review or meta-analysis, and how to apply results of these exercises in clinical practice.

Qualitative research methodology is the subject of Chapter 4. Key characteristics of, and ethical issues in, qualitative research are described. Purposive sampling strategies are summarized, and much attention is paid to comparing and evaluating the different approaches to gathering, preparing and analysing qualitative data. Methods of presenting qualitative research findings are discussed, and criteria for evaluating the quality of qualitative research are suggested last.

Chapters 5 and 6 relate to minimizing survey errors, while noting that the same errors also characterize other quantitative study designs. Chapter 5 describes a taxonomy of survey errors. It discusses, in turn, the main types of these errors and how, in particular, to minimize the occurrence of sampling error and the (non-observation) errors that can result when all or some intended measurements cannot be made on some part of the target population or sample. Chapter 6 focuses on how to minimize the different observation errors of measurement and processing in survey research.

Chapter 7 considers randomized controlled trials. It discusses ethical considerations and limitations of this study design before describing stages of clinical trials and evaluating ways of classifying randomized trial designs. The chapter then offers guidance on estimating sample sizes for randomized trials, on what to include in reporting these trials and on how to apply trial findings.

The final chapter, Chapter 8, offers practical advice on how to plan, write and publish health research. After discussing the steps involved in these processes, it focuses attention on how to write clear, concise and effective prose, and how to produce effective tables, graphs and maps. The chapter concludes by summarizing evidence on how to transfer research to the target audience.

REFERENCES

[1]   Miles M, Huberman A. *Qualitative Data Analysis: A Sourcebook of New Methods.* Beverly Hills, CA: Sage, 1994.

Chapter 1

CONCEPTUALIZING THE RESEARCH JOURNEY

OBJECTIVES

By the time you have completed this chapter, you should be able to:

1. Describe the major types of research.
2. Understand the concept of paradigms
3. Describe the nature, purpose and different levels of theory
4. Discuss different metatheories.
5. Match different types of research question to different metatheories and methodologies
6. Compare inductive and deductive theory as routes to reasoning and explanation
7. Compare and contrast qualitative, quantitative and mixed methods research
8. Consider ethical issues in health research

PREVIEW

This chapter explores influential approaches to producing knowledge and understanding as foundations for health research and social change. It begins by summarizing different types of research, which are each conceptualized to constitute a journey requiring a roadmap. To help us find a roadmap that can take us toward where we want to go, the chapter refers to systems of patterned beliefs that organize behavior. These take into account levels of theory, which help us to reflect critically on where we 'fit' with respect to the belief systems. Different research methodologies are also shown to be underpinned by the belief systems. Lastly, the chapter looks at general approaches to reasoning and explanation in different types of research; compares characteristics of quantitative, qualitative and mixed methods research; and reviews some of the fundamental ethical issues influencing health research.

TYPES OF RESEARCH

In this book, we will take a journey together – a journey that considers both how to critically use existing health research and how to produce our own health research. For the purpose of this journey, research can be defined as a careful and thorough investigation or inquiry, which is undertaken to solve problems, consider ideas and increase knowledge and understanding. Table 1.1 suggests one way to define the main types and purposes of research.

Table 1.1. Pasteur's Quadrant [1]

		Considerations of usefulness	
		Low	High
Quest for fundamental understanding	Yes	Pure basic research (e.g. Bohr) produces fundamental knowledge as an end in itself	Use-inspired basic research (e.g. Pasteur) produces fundamental knowledge of potential relevance to real world problems in specified broad areas
	No	Research that is self-serving (e.g. publishing for the sake of publishing)	Pure applied research (e.g. Edison) produces practical knowledge or change, of value to society as quickly as possible

Pure applied research can be conceptualized as taking at least three forms:

1. Research and Development to discover knowledge and recommend change,
2. Action research to solve a real world problem and act for improvement, and
3. Evaluation research to judge an intervention against a standard and give feedback.

Table 1.2. Typology of Evaluation Research

Formative evaluation to identify ongoing opportunities, during the development phase, to improve an intervention and inform decision-making	• Needs assessment to assess needs and how they may be best met • Process evaluation to assess whether the intervention is being implemented as intended
Summative evaluation to assess the effects or outcomes of the intervention against its stated goals	• Outcome evaluation to assess outcomes immediately once the implementation of the intervention ends • Impact evaluation to assess effects of the intervention as a whole over the long-term • Economic evaluation to compare benefits and costs of the intervention

The subject of evaluation research lies largely outside the scope of this book. Nevertheless, some of the research methods we will cover are applicable to this type of applied research. Table 1.2 summarizes key types of formative evaluation and summative evaluation. Stakes has been quoted by Patton (p. 69) [2] as offering a clear and memorable distinction between these types: 'When the cook tastes the soup, that's formative. When the guests taste the soup, that's summative.'

PARADIGMS

Research is a journey towards knowledge and understanding. However, its search for understanding, according to the German philosopher Hans-Georg Gadamer (and in his latter work, Ludwig Wittgenstein), is an ongoing and emergent process that may change with time and never be completed. In common with Schubert's 8th and 9th symphonies, it may be described as 'Unfinished' and 'Incomplete' respectively. This journey is worth taking because of the splendid sights along the way, sights that enable us at least to approximate truth and achieve truth-likeness (verisimilitude).

To take our journey, we need a 'roadmap' to help direct or guide us. A 'paradigm' meets this need. It is a patterned, shared way of viewing the world which organizes the set of practices that define a discipline during a particular time period. Paradigms have at least four critical features. They are impossible to compare in value (incommensurable); are untestable; provide alternative ways of seeing and understanding; and are slow to change.

In health research, examples of paradigms are the 'particle' paradigm and 'social' paradigm [3]. The particle paradigm focuses on people as individuals. Conspicuously through the lenses of medicine and psychology, it sees them respectively as organisms and psychological beings. In contrast, the social paradigm views people primarily in terms of their social relationships [3].

NATURE, PURPOSE AND LEVELS OF THEORY

Key elements of any paradigm are (1) basic elements (including a disciplinary matrix of basic and strongly held beliefs, values and assumptions), (2) theory, (3) exemplars (shared concrete solutions to substantive problems) and (4) methodology. A methodology is the interlocking rules or principles that describe and prescribe a plan of the methods that are available and acceptable to help explore the world as theory defines it. Methods are the procedures, tools or techniques used to generate and analyze data. To understand the role of 'theory' in paradigms, Table 1.3 defines theory, explains its importance and influence on research and then describes four ordered levels of theory that can characterize paradigms and research.

Table 1.3. Finding Direction from Theory

What is theory?	• Theory provides a set of ideas or statements for conceptually exploring something. It may range from supposition to explicit hypotheses
Why is theory important?	• Theory gives direction to where we are going. It is also like a lens that we can look through to see the world clearly. Our choice of theory influences what questions we pose, how we answer them and what the results mean or signify. It can be used to describe, explain, predict, prescribe or even control what we suppose or observe in the world
How does theory influence research?	• Theory gives direction by using concepts to structure our attempts to view the world and make sense of the things we find

Level of theory	Name of level	Characteristics	Example
Highest, most abstract level	Metatheory (theory about theory)	• The most global theory • Very abstract and more fundamental than other theories • Not testable empirically but embraces lower levels of theory	Logical positivism
	Grand theory	• Highly abstract, comprehensive and widely applicable • Comprises general concepts and makes broad generalizations • Counterintuitive, offering a novel perspective • Cannot be tested empirically	Psychoanalytic theory
	Middle range theory	• Sufficiently abstract to be scientifically interesting • Focuses on limited aspects of social organization and behavior • Easily applicable in practice and directly testable • Limited number of variables, and so conceptually economic	Health belief model
Lowest, least abstract level	Micro (practice) theory	• Hypotheses about narrowly defined phenomena • Suggests prescriptions or modalities for practice • Concrete and easily tested empirically	Turn and reposition bed-ridden patients often to prevent pressure ulcers

What is the scale of the different maps (level of the theory)?

What is the scale of the different maps (level of the theory)?

Table 1.4. Metatheories as Routes to Explanation

Issue	Metatheory					
	Logical positivism	Post-positivism	Pragmatism	Constructivism/ interpretivism/ naturalism	Critical theory	Participatory
Aim	• Verify hypotheses • Uncover truths (facts or causes) • Explain and predict events	• Infer from non-falsified hypotheses what is probably true	• Define the meaning or truth of ideas through the practical results of their use • Produce current, workable solutions of real-world problems	• Mentally construct an understanding of (i.e. interpret) some social phenomenon from the meaning that it has to those with lived experience of it in specific contexts	• Critique Transcend social conditions to expose hidden interests and contradictions • Transform and emancipate society	• Practical knowing and action for human flourishing
Assumed nature of reality (ontology)	• Naïve realism/ common sense realism • There is an objectively knowable, mind-independent reality. We can know how things are, either from direct appeal to the senses (empiricism; the 'positivist' part) or, by inferring from sense-experience, explicit sequences of steps to produce a particular result (the 'logical' part)	• Critical realism • There is an objective, external reality that can be approximated but not fully understood. So, what we perceive must undergo the widest possible scrutiny	• Subtle realism • An objective reality exists. It is represented tentatively, probabilistically and always from a particular perspective. Reality is also understood in terms of the consequences of belief, and by what is necessary to produce the outcome intended	• Relativism • Different worldviews give rise to multiple subjective realities. • Truth does not correspond with an objective reality. It is co-constructed by the interactions that take place between the researcher and what is researched	• Historical/ material realism • For critical theorists, social reality is socially constructed through consensus. The truth is hidden by a reified, 'virtual' reality	• Participative reality • There is a 'subjective-objective' reality, which is one co-created by our minds and the world

Table 1.4 (Continued)

Issue	Logical positivism	Post-positivism	Pragmatism	Constructivism	Critical theory	Participatory
Assumed nature of relationship between knower and known (epistemology)	• Certainty is objectively possible (epistemological absolutism) • Separation of the knower (the subject) and the known (the object) (dualism)	• Knowers differ in their understandings of what is probably objectively real (epistemological relativism) • Dualism is not possible	• Negotiated provisionally through experience and reason, knowledge is what works or not in actual practice • Transactions between human agents and their environment replace the knower-known distinction	• The knower is at one with the known (no extra-mental reality) • The ontological-epistemological distinction thus dissolves; what is really there and the (fused) relation of the knower-known are different versions of the same question	• Knowledge is what enables emancipation through changing values that make material differences. It is revealed through critical thought and discussion	• Knower participates in the known through different ways of knowing, including practical knowing • These produce the challenge to be critically subjective
Assumed role of values in inquiry (axiology)	• Value-free	• Values are present but their influence can be controlled	• Values strongly influence interpretation	• Value-bound	• Value-mediated	• Value-mediated
Plan of the methods we can use to explore the world (methodology)	• Quantitative research • Observes and measures to verify hypotheses as facts or laws, which correspond with the real world	• Quantitative and qualitative research • Uses methods to replicate findings that are probably true but always falsifiable	• Quantitative and qualitative research • Uses the methods (including mixed methods) best able to answer the question posed in each situation	• Qualitative research • Describes and interprets patterns of meaning in their natural contexts	• Dialogic and dialectical analysis • Historical revisionism	• Cooperative inquiry • Participants have the right to participate fully in the research, which is grounded in experience

Table 1.4 (Continued)

Issue	Logical positivism	Post-positivism	Pragmatism	Constructivism	Critical theory	Participatory
Examples of methodologies can be:	• Experiments and other deductive methodologies that seek to show a correspondence with the real world	• Deductive methodologies • Inductive approaches, e.g. grounded theory (early statements)	• Mixed methodologies	• Grounded theory (later statements) • Symbolic interactionism • Hermeneutic phenomenology • Discourse analysis	• Critical theory • Deconstruction	• Participatory action research
Characteristics	• Deductive • Logical • Deterministic • Reductionist • Structured • Mechanistic • Precise	• Theory-laden • Structured • Probabilistic • Fallibilistic	• Deductive, inductive and abductive • Action-focused • Holistic • Contextual • Outcome-oriented • Instrumentalist • Compatibilist	• Inductive • Holistic • Flexible	• Dialogic • Critical • Practical • Collaborative • Emancipatory	• Participatory • Experiential • Collaborative • Political • Practical • Self-reflexive
Criteria for assessment	• Internal validity • External validity • Reliability • Objectivity		• Workability (predictability and applicability)	• Credibility • Transferability • Dependability • Confirmability	• Theoretical consistency • Historical insights • Emancipatory implications	• Human flourishing

Table 1.5. Central Questions and Methods associated with Different Metatheories

Metatheory • Methodology	Central question	Principal methods
Positivism	What logically deduced hypotheses can be verified empirically?	
• Logical positivism	• What is the truth in the real world?	• Experimentation, manipulation, measurement
• Ethnography	• What are the cultural understandings and meanings that this group constructs as its members carry out their daily lives?	• Intensive fieldwork: extended, participant observation; informal depth interviews; and note-taking
Post-positivism	Which rival hypotheses are more or less plausible and valid?	
• Classical grounded theory	• What theory can be constructed from, and in relation to, the information gathered in order to account for observations made? • How can the veils hiding reality be lifted?	Theoretical sampling, depth interviewing, observation, constant comparison
Pragmatism	What is the most appropriate solution to this real-world problem?	Mixed methods: quantitative and qualitative
Constructivism	How do people's constructions of social reality influence their behavior?	
• Symbolic interactionism	• What common symbols and understandings give shared meaning to, and influence, social interactions?	Group interviews
• Ethnomethodology	• How do people make sense of their everyday life to maintain the social order?	• 'Ethnomethodological experiments' that may disrupt everyday activity; participant observation; depth interviews
• Phenomenology	• What is the *essential* nature of some phenomenon, which gives it the meaning that lives within people's conscious experience?	• Depth interviews. Disinterested reduction of pre-reflective descriptions of direct experience to their essential meaning. • Depth interviews.
• Hermeneutic phenomenology	• What is the hidden, *existential* meaning of some phenomenon, which lives within everyday experience?	The researcher grows an interpretation from analysis of conversations that acknowledge the biases and presuppositions of each participant in situated reflection
Critical theory	How can the ways in which power and injustice shape people's experiences be understood and used to change society?	
• Feminisms	• How does the lens of gender shape human relationships and social processes? How can women's knowledge be liberating?	Participatory and collaborative processes
• Cultural studies	• How do historical and social structures and discourses shape how contemporary culture is lived and changes?	Textual analysis as criticism: literary/critical techniques; ethnography
• Postmodernism	• How does language shape the social construction of the dominant group and not represent reality fully?	Discourse analysis, deconstruction (Derrida), genealogical method (Foucault)
• Participatory inquiry	• How can individuals be enabled to flourish?	Inquiry methods agreed on by the researcher and participants

METATHEORY

Table 1.3 introduced the concept of metatheory. Meta-theories are the general theoretical part of paradigms, describing and prescribing a vision of what is acceptable as a theory of first principles in a scientific discipline. The prefix 'meta-' means 'about' (its category). So, metatheories are theories about theories. Metatheories are smaller than paradigms because, as noted above, paradigms also include the basic elements, methodologies and exemplars closely related to metatheories.

Which metatheory should we choose? No one metatheory is necessarily always the best. Each of us must decide for ourselves which metatheory to use (and when) on the basis of how we individually view the world. However, this chapter can help us to decide by scrutinizing the claims (about issues such as the nature of reality) that different metatheories make. This scrutiny is also important because lack of awareness of how metatheory shapes people's research can lead to questionable attempts to link some methodologies to each other or to particular questions. Table 1.4 compares five metatheories (and related methodologies). Table 1.5 states key questions and methods associated with these metatheories.

DEDUCTION AND INDUCTION

Different metatheories and methodologies may be mainly deductive, mainly inductive, or both (Table 1.4). The terms, 'deductive' and 'inductive' require explanation. They can refer to the form of logic used in making arguments (a system of claims, or statements, one of which is supported by the others) (Table 1.6) as well as to the route taken to achieve explanation or understanding (see Table 1.7). The different routes to explanation describe and prescribe overlapping methodologies for creating knowledge in order to explain, predict, understand and control phenomena. These methodologies – including the inductive method and the hypothetico-deductive method – give rise to inductive confirmation, through the probability of a theory being true, and to deductive falsification through 'conjectures and refutations.' Other conceptualizations include 'progressive research programmes' that are better than others rather than necessarily true or false. Research can thus advance science through evolutionary change or, when enough significant anomalies cannot be explained by a current paradigm, through a revolutionary shift to a new, 'better' paradigm.

QUANTITATIVE AND QUALITATIVE RESEARCH

The terms quantitative and qualitative are adjectives commonly attached to, or imposed on, the methodologies and methods used in health research. Quantitative and qualitative research methodologies, and mixed methods research, are important vehicles for traveling along the routes we are taking toward knowledge and understanding. Table 1.8 compares general characteristics of quantitative and qualitative research, but risks some over-simplification in its aim for clarity.

Table 1.6. Deductive and Inductive Arguments

	Deductive argument	Inductive argument
Definition	Determines what *must* be true *if* the premises (starting assumptions) are true; hence it can offer absolute certainty	• Generalizes from *some* observations or evidence to what is *probably* true if the premises are true; hence it can offer only probability
Purpose	Make predictions about an hypothesis (which can be tested via induction); transmit and preserve the truth	• Generate hypotheses and theory; discover the truth
Basic form	If P then Q If Q then R Therefore, if P then R	Every P I have seen is Q These are Ps Therefore these Ps are Q

Other forms		• Other forms [4] include abduction (or abductive induction):
		  There is Q
		    If P then Q-
		    Therefore, probably P
		• This has appeal to pragmatists by starting with the consequent, Q, and reasoning back to the best (most probable) explanation: that Q is caused by P. In so doing, it makes an inference about an 'unobservable' and allows for the possibility of better explanations than P. The 'inductive inferences' of grounded theory may be best described as 'abductive' [5].

Precautions	Form-dependent Before testing the conclusion, R, check for ambiguity in the premises and whether the conclusion follows logically and necessarily from them.	• Content-dependent • Check the truth of the claims, account for all relevant information and ensure the inference is properly made
Property of truth	Applies to the claims of an argument and their correspondence with an external reality (correspondence theory) or each other (coherence theory); some dispute these concepts of truth and offer alternative (e.g. pragmatic) conceptualizations.	
Property of validity	Describes the whole of a deductive argument (see Chapter 5)	• Inductive arguments are better or worse, not valid or invalid

Table 1.7. Routes to Explanation

Place of theory	Mainly deductive, top-down approach (e.g. Scientific method)	Mainly inductive, bottom-up approach (e.g. 'Baconian' route to explanation; classical grounded theory [6])	Mixed deductive-inductive approach (e.g. Grounded theory of Strauss and Corbin [7]; analytic induction)
Theory driven / Theory testing	Review existing literature Select topic Select theory Develop hypotheses Deduce 'facts' that follow from the hypotheses Test the truth of the facts through observation or by conducting an experiment Confirm or disconfirm the hypothesis, thereby helping to test the theory		Select topic Identify orienting theory Develop working hypotheses Test hypotheses, e.g. through constant comparison of the theory and data, including initial categories, negative cases (see Table 4.7) and reviewed literature
Data driven / Theory generation/ theory building		Undertake observation Generate theory from consistent results Identify patterns. Compare categories with each other and with reviewed literature Infer emergent and tentative theory	Modify the hypotheses until all the cases fit. Refine the theory

Table 1.8. Characteristics of Quantitative and Qualitative Research

Quantitative research	Qualitative research
Aims to describe the study phenomenon and predict causal relationships through reduction, control, precision and explanation	Aims to understand the meaning of human action from different perspectives through detailed description and shared interpretation
Assumes an objective reality, which is separate from the researcher and may or may not be understood fully or always in the same way	Varies in its assumptions about the nature of reality and emphasizes subjective, lived experience as the source of our knowledge
Attempts to remove or control the effect of the values and interests of researchers on their work	Tends to see researchers' values as helping to guide and shape their research
Tends to focus narrowly on selected, predefined variables and investigate how these interact	Tends to focus contextually on the whole situation under study as greater than the parts
Emphasizes the use of deductive reasoning to provide evidence for or against prespecified hypotheses, and test known theory; but quantitative research can also be exploratory	Emphasizes the use of inductive or dialectical reasoning, e.g. to generate hypotheses or develop theory; however, qualitative research can also involve deductive analysis and be confirmatory
Predetermines structured study designs, which may manipulate the study conditions	Produces flexible, emergent and evolving study designs that favor natural settings for research
Reviews literature early in the study	Reviews literature review as the study progresses or afterwards
Prefers to sample subjects randomly, considers sample size important and is dedicated to generalization on the basis of statistical inference	Samples participants purposively, considers the richness of the sample most important, and uses logical inference to assess results' transferability
Emphasizes the collection of numeric data, statistical analysis and measurable outcomes	Emphasizes the collection and analysis of non-numeric data in the form of words
Uses inanimate instruments	Uses communication and observation; the researcher is the primary collection instrument

MULTI-METHOD, MIXED-METHOD, AND MIXED-MODEL RESEARCH

Some researchers, such as Denzin and Lincoln [8], are philosophical purists. Reflecting their particular view of the world, they avoid mixing meta-theories, methodologies and methods whose underlying premises they consider incompatible. However, many (if not most) researchers operate not at the poles but near the center. For example, Patton [9] avoids adhering to any named meta-theory. His research is largely question and methods driven. Such researchers mix methodologies when:

1. The methodologies share the same ontological foundation. Within an individual study, these methodologies are probably best used as discrete, separate approaches (to maintain their integrity) [10]. For example, 'transcendental phenomenology' and 'classical grounded theory' assume critical realist ontologies. In contrast, 'hermeneutic phenomenology' and Strauss and Corbin's version of grounded theory both assume relativist ontologies.
2. The methodologies, even when they make different assumptions about the nature of reality and knowledge, provide a way of filtering different elements from complex and uncertain wholes, enabling us to see the world through different lenses in response to our particular and changing needs and questions [11]. This pragmatic approach focuses on what can be useful. For example, it may be appropriate at different times to name and count errors (positivism), look for hidden explanations (critical theory) or interactively co-create an innovative plan to manage the errors (constructivism).
3. A single meta-theory combines insights from other meta-theories. For example, 'pragmatism and critical theory have qualities of post-positivism and interpretivism' [12] (p. 5).

Sometimes a distinction is also made between multi-method research, mixed method research, and mixed model research.

Multi-method research (intra-method mixing) refers to mixing methods within qualitative or quantitative research; for example, using questionnaires that contain open and closed questions.

Mixed-method research (inter-method mixing) refers to mixing qualitative and quantitative research methods in studies that use the same methodology (as in pragmatism) or different methodologies. In the latter situation, different typologies of mixed-method research [13-15] highlight dimensions such as (1) time order – whether the methods of each methodology are used in parallel or sequentially; (2) methodology emphasis – whether each methodology has equal status or not; and (3) the purpose of mixing methods (e.g. exploration, explanation, triangulation or transformation).

Mixed model research: This mixes quantitative and qualitative methods within or across stages of the research, frequently to answer qualitative and quantitative research questions.

How can we decide whether to mix methods? The methods used should always be driven by the research question and whether we believe that different methods can, given their different assumptions and theoretical starting points, be sensibly and usefully combined. Table 1.9 compares strengths and weaknesses of research using qualitative, quantitative and mixed methods respectively.

Table 1.9. Strengths and Weaknesses of Quantitative, Qualitative and Mixed Methods Research

	Quantitative research	Qualitative research	Mixed methods research
Strengths	Can test and help to validate existing and new hypotheses and theories	Can answer questions about the meanings of findings	Combines methodological strengths of quantitative and qualitative research
	Can answer questions about event frequency and rate, and about effect size	Can produce understanding of how and why events occur	Can address an expanded range of research questions
	Can establish causal relationships and predict future events quantitatively	Can develop theory	Can use methods with complementary strengths and non-overlapping weaknesses to offer a picture of increased completeness
	Is rigorous, can minimize bias, and yields precise, often replicable findings	Can reflect multiple perspectives, including participants' experiences, viewpoints and priorities	Can use triangulation to enhance the credibility, confirmability and transferrability of results
	Can permit generalizations to target populations	Can detail descriptions and study cases in depth	
	Is credible with key decision-makers	Yields naturalistic data, aiding data transfer	
	Can base conclusions on the analysis of large amounts of data	Can respond to changes occurring during the study	
	Can permit the collection and analysis of data to occur relatively fast	Can study cases in context	
		Can provide detailed information on individual cases, including what causes particular events	
		Can permit cross-case comparison and analysis	
Weaknesses	Can yield results with which local participants disagree	Has an increased potential for (disabling) researcher bias	Can waste effort on duplicating findings
	Focus on confirmation, rather than generation, of theories or hypotheses (confirmation bias)	Can be difficult to generalize to other people or settings	Mixes paradigms and can easily violate methodological assumptions of each method
	Produces aggregated results that can be difficult to apply to individual cases	Can be time consuming and comparatively expensive	Is unclear on how to manage inconsistent findings
	Is ill-suited to investigating complex and unpredictable human behavior	Tends to lack credibility with key decision-makers, including funders	Is ambiguous on how best to mix the methods
			Has not clearly indicated how to analyze quantitative data qualitatively, and vice versa
			Can require a research team with skills in both using and mixing both methodologies
			Can be costly in money and time

ETHICS

The most important moral safeguard is 'the presence of an intelligent, informed, conscientious, compassionate, responsible investigator' [16]. However, we must also ensure that our proposed research methods undergo ethics review by an independent ethics committee (institutional review board) and satisfy its ethical requirements. Ethics committees cannot relieve us of the responsibility to think through the ethical implications of our intended research. But they can provide a 'safety net' in making concrete decisions based most commonly on the specification, at least implicitly, of abstract principles of secular ethics to suit each particular case (principlism).

Each of the principles, on face value, is binding unless it conflicts with another ethical principle whereupon a balanced choice is required between them. Table 1.10 describes the four principles of medical ethics developed by Beauchamp and Childress [17]. An attraction of these principles is their connection to a common morality. However, limitations of principlism have led to calls for alternative or supplementary ethical systems, such as those based on a supreme principle or an ethic based in virtue, caring, 'experience' or the cases themselves (casuistry) [18].

Table 1.10. Ethical Principles in Health Research

Principle	Definition	Consequent need for the research to:
Non-maleficence	Avoid doing harm to others	• Minimize risks • Protect people's physical and cultural safety • Compensate for harm • Ensure research adequacy
Beneficence	Prevent harm, and do good	• Be able to reasonably expect that the benefits to the public good will outweigh the risks
Autonomy	Respect the self-determination of competent persons	• Consult with individuals and groups • Obtain informed and voluntary consent • Respect people's privacy • Protect people's confidentiality and anonymity • Limit the use of deception
Justice	Fairly distribute benefits, risks and costs	• Select subjects/participants fairly

REFERENCES

[1]   Stokes D. *Pasteur's quadrant. Basic Science and Technological Innovation.* Washington DC: Brookings Institution Press, 1997.

[2]   Patton M. *Utilization-focused Evaluation: The New Century Text.* 3rd Edition. Thousand Oaks: Sage, 1997.

[3]   Adams P. *Fragmented Intimacy: Addiction in a Social World.* New York: Springer, In press.

[4]   Demeterio FI. Logic, the philosophy of systematic thinking and argumentation. *Diwatao* 2001;1(1). *http://www.geocities.com/philodept/diwatao/logic.htm*

[5]   Baggini J, Fosl P. *The Philosopher's Toolkit. A Compendium of Philosophical Concepts and Methods*. Oxford: Blackwell Publishing, 2003.

[6]   Glaser B. *Basics of Grounded Theory Analysis*. California: Sociology Press, 1992.

[7]   Strauss A, Corbin J. *Basics of Qualitative Research*. California: Sage Publications, 1990.

[8]   Denzin N, Lincoln Y (eds). *The Sage Handbook of Qualitative Research*. Thousand Oaks: Sage Publications, 2005.

[9]   Patton M. *Qualitative Research and Evaluation Methods*. Thousand Oaks: Sage Publications, 2002.

[10]   Annells M. Triangulation of qualitative approaches: hermeneutical phenomenology and grounded theory. *J Adv Nurs* 2006;56:55-61.

[11]   Thomas P. General medical practitioners need to be aware of the theories on which our work depends. *Ann Fam Med* 2006;4:450-4.

[12]   Miles M, Huberman A. *Qualitative Data Analysis: A Sourcebook of New Methods*. Beverly Hills, CA: Sage, 1994.

[13]   Cresswell J. *Research Design: Qualitative, Quantitative and Mixed Methods Approaches*. 2nd Edition. Thousand Oaks, CA: Sage, 2003.

[14]   Tashakkori A, Teddlie C. The past and future of mixed methods research from data triangulation to mixed model designs. In: Tashakkori A, Teddlie C (eds). *Handbook of Mixed Methods in the Social and Behavioural Sciences*. Thousand Oaks, CA: Sage, 2003.

[15]   Johnson B, Onwuegbuzie A. Mixed methods research: A research paradigm whose time has come. *Educ Res* 2004;33:14-26.

[16]   Beecher H. Ethics and clinical research. *N Eng J Med* 1966;274:367-72.

[17]   Beauchamp TL, Childress JF. *Principles of Biomedical Ethics*. 5th Edition. Oxford: Oxford University Press, 2001.

[18]   Pellegrino E. The metamorphosis of medical ethics: A 30-year retrospective. *JAMA* 1993;269:1158-62.

Chapter 2

STUDY QUESTIONS, STUDY DESIGNS AND STUDY MEASURES

OBJECTIVES

By the time you have completed this chapter, you should be able to:

1. Formulate a good research question or aims, objectives and any hypotheses
2. Compare major study designs for answering different research questions
3. Describe and calculate basic measures of frequency and effect
4. Demonstrate understanding of the statistical concepts of p values and confidence intervals

PREVIEW

This chapter helps to set the foundations for constructing and using good health research. It considers how to ask a good research question, before focusing on how to select the most feasible study design (a) to answer questions suited to quantitative research and (b) to bridge the quantitative-qualitative research divide. The chapter then discusses how to calculate and interpret across quantitative study designs some of the key measures of frequency and common measures of the effect of particular exposures (including potential risk factors, diagnostic tests, and treatments).

GOOD RESEARCH QUESTIONS

A research question specifies explicitly what we want to study. Individual studies typically focus on one question, or a small number. Generating good research questions is a creative process that tends to reflect how we view the world (Chapter 1) and can require experience, intuition, imagination and inductive reasoning. It can also lead to, and be refined by, a meaningful literature review.

I like research questions that challenge assumptions which other people take for granted. But iconoclastic challenges to the status quo require strong defensible arguments, since they will almost certainly encounter resistance. The new arguments may be found through a re-examination of the premises supporting existing arguments. Table 2.1 describes some approaches to doing this. It covers inductive methods (canons) of causal reasoning that can be used to generate questions about cause and effect [1]. These methods reflect the work of the philosopher and economist, John Stuart Mill.

Table 2.1. Methods of Causal Reasoning

Name	Formula	Example
Method of agreement	A and B occur with Y and Z A and C occur with X and Z So probably A is the cause of Z	• Among patients who developed particular symptoms, all had one thing in common: they had eaten chicken from the same establishment. So, we have reason to ask the research question: did eating contaminated chicken produce the symptoms? Or to hypothesize that eating the chicken caused the symptoms
Method of difference	A and B occur with Y and Z B occurs with Y So probably A is the cause of Z	• Only those who ate the chicken fell ill, so we could posit the same question or hypothesis as stated above
Joint method of agreement and difference	A and B occur with Y and Z A and B occur with Y and Z A and C occur with X and Z B occurs with Y So probably A is the cause of Z	• Combination of the first two methods
Method of residue	A and B occur with Y and Z B is previously known to be a cause of Y So probably A is the cause of Z	• If everyone who fell ill also ate canned foods, but it is known that contaminated canned foods produce different symptoms, we may ask whether, or hypothesize that, chicken caused the current outbreak of suspected food poisoning
Method of concomitant variation	Change in A, then Z also changes. So probably A is the cause of Z	• The more chicken that people ate, the worse their illness symptoms. So we may ask or hypothesize whether symptom severity is proportional to the amount of infected chicken eaten

Much research fails to advance knowledge, not because it is technically flawed but because the question posed is poor. Good research questions are clear, usually simple, and specific. They are also feasible to 'answer,' relevant, interesting and, within reason, original. They state the purposes and context of the research. It is important therefore to take the time to get the question right.

In qualitative research, the question may evolve as the study progresses. Creswell [2] offers some useful guidelines for writing qualitative research questions. For example, he recommends that researchers state one or two central questions in a general form, followed by associated subquestions. All these questions typically begin with 'what' or 'how,' use active verbs indicative of the research methodology, focus on a single concept or phenomenon, and mention the participants.

Focused from the outset, quantitative research questions are questions that the researcher intends to answer, not merely investigate. They commonly focus on describing variables, examining relationships between variables or determining differences between the study groups on selected variables. One approach to setting a good question for quantitative health research is PECOT (see below) [3]. Besides providing a GATE (Graphic Appraisal Tool for Epidemiological studies) for 'hanging' and appraising studies, it requires that questions (and appraisals) specify, as relevant, the:

Participants
Exposure group (e.g. allocated to an intervention or exposed to a risk factor)
Comparison (control) group
Outcome(s)
Time (at one point in time or over a period of time)

For example, are beta-blockers better than diuretics at lowering 5-year cardiovascular risk in patients over the age of 50 with hypertension but without other disease

---

Participants = patients aged > 50 years with diagnosed high blood pressure
Exposure = beta-blockers
Comparison group = diuretics
Outcome = cardiovascular disease events
Time = five years

STUDY AIMS, OBJECTIVES AND HYPOTHESES

A research question can be presented as the study *aim*, which states what the study is intending to achieve. In the example above, the aim is to compare the effectiveness of beta-blockers and diuretics in reducing cardiovascular risk in patients over age 50 with hypertension but not other disease. In contrast, our study *objective* is what we are proposing to deliver in order to achieve this aim (e.g. the objective is to produce experimental evidence of the effectiveness of each treatment in the study population).

Qualitative researchers prefer research questions to objectives written as specific goals [2]. Moreover, in quantitative research, objectives may be presented as (or lead to) *hypotheses* that state provisionally, and either directionally or non-directionally, what we are expecting the study to show (e.g. that there is no difference in the effectiveness of the treatments in our study population).

According to Popper [4], hypotheses must also be falsifiable to be scientific. Not all research requires hypotheses to test. As Table 1.8 noted, qualitative research, for example, tends to be hypothesis-generating. However, much quantitative research develops and tests hypotheses based on some intuitive 'picturing' of how the world is structured. Produced at the outset of the study, hypotheses can give a clear focus and predetermine the probability of a specific result occurring.

STUDY DESIGNS

The broad strategy for answering research questions (and testing any hypotheses) is known as the study design (or study plan). The purpose of Figure 2.1 and Tables 2.2 and 2.3 is to help us select the study design that can best answer our research questions when these are suited to quantitative research, within the resources available. However, Table 2.4 summarizes two other sets of approaches – case study designs and historical-comparative study designs – which can bridge quantitative and qualitative research. Qualitative research has resisted the need for precise study designs, and tended to present them as methodologies. (see Chapter 4 and Table 1.5).

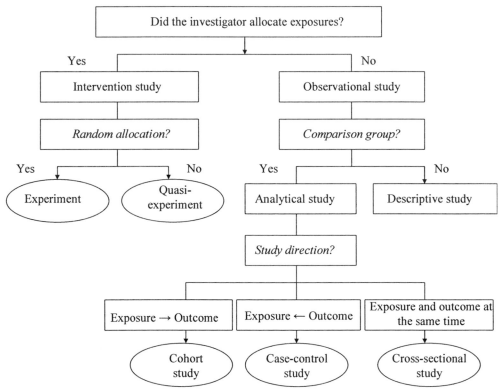

Figure 2.1. Interventional and Observational Study Designs.
Reprinted (with small changes) from The Lancet, Vol. 359, Grimes DA, Schulz KF, An overview of clinical research: the lay of the land, 57-61, Copyright 5 January 2002, with permission from Elsevier.

Intervention Studies

Table 2.2 focuses on designs for evaluating interventions. In these studies the researcher allocates the exposure, i.e. intervenes. Intervention studies aim to answer research questions about whether the intervention 'works;' for example, whether it is effective. The allocation of interventions may be randomized (made random) or non-randomized. Chapter 7 elaborates on randomized trials. For non-randomized studies, Table 2.2. can be used in conjunction with the TREND (Transparent Reporting of Evaluations with Non-randomized Designs) Statement for improving the quality of reporting [5].

Table 2.2. Study Designs for Evaluating Interventions

Type	Subtype	Description	Graphical representation	Objectives	Advantages	Disadvantages
			R = random allocation X_E = study intervention X_C = control intervention O = measurement. Left to right dimension indicates temporal sequence			
Experiment (randomized design)	Randomized controlled trial (RCT) (includes single patient trials and crossover trials)	Directly compares the impact of the 'experimental intervention' and the 'control intervention' on participants randomized to each group	Group A R ----- O ----- X_E ----- O Group B R ----- O ----- X_C ----- O	Test effect of the experimental intervention against the control intervention	Unbiased distribution of confounders	Expensive Volunteer bias Potential for poor external validity. Can be ethically problematic
Quasi-experiment (non-randomized design) [6 7]	Time series study (with or without a control group)	Compares performance at multiple time points both before and after the intervention. (Any control group (Group B) does not receive this intervention)	Group A O --- O --- X --- O --- O (Group B O --- O --- O --- O --- O)	Test whether the effect of the intervention is greater than any underlying secular trend	Useful when it is difficult to randomize or identify an appropriate control group	Need data on multiple time points before and after the intervention

Table 2.2 (Continued)

Type	Subtype	Description	Graphical representation	Objectives	Advantages	Disadvantages
	Simple before and after study (with or without a control group); this is a special case of the time series design	Compares performance measured once before and once after the intervention. (Any control group (Group B) does not receive this intervention)	Group A O -------- X -------- O (Group B O -------- O -------- O)	Same as randomized controlled trial	Compared with randomized trials, more feasible and less expensive for large studies	Lack of randomization threatens the internal validity of the study through selection bias. Secular trends or sudden changes can make it difficult to attribute observed changes to the intervention

Observational Studies

Table 2.3 summarizes designs for observational studies [8]. In these studies the investigator observes the effect of exposures on the outcome of interest, without allocating or manipulating these exposures. Observational studies can answer questions about the occurrence and distribution of outcomes, and test hypotheses about observed effects of the exposures ('natural' treatments). The table relates specific observational study designs to certain types of questions.

Study Designs Bridging the Quantitative-Qualitative Divide

The foregoing study designs are associated mainly with quantitative research in which *variables* and measurement take center stage. In contrast, the following two sets of study designs focus on *cases* and claim to avoid the excesses associated with other, more rigid methodologies.

1. *Case studies* examine, in detail, cases as bounded (in place and time), concrete and specific instances of a phenomenon selected for study [9]. There are competing conceptualizations of case study designs. However, following Yin [10], case studies draw on multiple sources of evidence, including quantitative or qualitative data, to investigate how or why contemporary phenomena (cases and their subunits) act as they do in their real-world contexts. These designs accommodate more variables of interest than data points, and benefit from theory development before the data collection and analysis. Table 2.4 summarizes basic design types for case studies [10 11]. Qualitative [12] and other typologies of case studies [13 14] have also been developed.
2. *Historical-comparative studies* variously use quantitative and qualitative research methods to compare whole cases in their specific, historical and/or cultural contexts. Researchers using this collection of approaches immerse themselves in diverse but limited data including their own perspectives. The purpose of doing this is to reconstruct from the evidence fragments the tentative understanding that is needed to translate situated systems of meaning into plausible, combinational and contingent accounts of the study phenomenon, and make limited generalizations [15].

Table 2.3. Observational Study Designs

Type	Subtype	Description	Graphical representation	Objectives	Advantages	Disadvantages
			C = Cases with event of interest; Ĉ = Non-cases; E = Exposure; Ē = Not exposed; N = population; S = Sample. Left to right dimension indicates temporal sequence			
Analytic studies	Cohort (longitudinal) study. Basic types are current prospective studies and retrospective (historical prospective) cohort studies	Follow individuals at risk of event (e.g. CVD) to see how many develop it given exposure or not to risk factors	N --- S --- Ĉ, with branches E → EĈ, EC and Ē → ĒĈ, ĒC	Make causal inferences about the risk of exposures producing new outcome(s) of interest	• Cheaper and easier than RCT • Can directly estimate incidence rates, and risks, for each exposure • Reduced bias in exposure measurement • Can test hypotheses and identify likely causes of common outcomes • Assess rare exposures	• No randomization • Often requires a large sample • More costly and time consuming than other observational studies • Historical cohort studies depend on record quality • Inefficient for rare outcomes • Potential for information bias, confounding and loss of subjects

Table 2.3 (Continued)

Type	Subtype	Description	Graphical representation	Objectives	Advantages	Disadvantages
	Case-control study	Compare cases (with outcome event of interest) and controls retrospectively with respect to exposures	$N \cdots C \begin{smallmatrix} \cdots \bar{E}C \\ \cdots EC \end{smallmatrix}$ $N \cdots S \cdots \hat{C} \begin{smallmatrix} \cdots \bar{E}\hat{C} \\ \cdots E\hat{C} \end{smallmatrix}$	• Test cause-effect hypotheses for specific rare event	• Can generate hypotheses • Ideal for new, rare events and those following a long lag after exposure • Can test multiple exposure hypotheses • Statistically efficient • Cheap, relatively easy and quick • Can detect short-term risks	• Cannot show cause-effect relationships • Cannot estimate incidence directly • Difficult to ensure the comparability of cases and controls • Potential for confounding, and selection and measurement biases • Not usually suited to investigating rare exposures • Single outcome is a binary variable

Table 2.3 (Continued)

Type	Subtype	Description	Graphical representation	Objectives	Advantages	Disadvantages
	Analytic cross-sectional study (sample survey)	Look for associations between common outcome and sample attributes measured at the same time	$N \text{ --- } S \text{ --- } \begin{cases} E\hat{C} \\ EC \\ \bar{E}\hat{C} \\ \bar{E}C \end{cases}$	• Identify possible cause and effect relationships • Generate and test hypotheses	• Best design to assess a diagnostic test • Ethically safe, cheap, quick and relatively easy to conduct • Can study many exposures and outcomes • Can measure prevalence and burden • Can be the basis of cohort studies	• At best can reveal common associations • Cannot estimate incidence; has the limitations of prevalences (Table 2.5) • Not suited to events that are rare or short-lived • Low response is a major threat; risk of recall bias
Descriptive studies	Descriptive cross-section al (point or period prevalence) study	Survey sample to estimate frequency of existing events of interest	As above	• Measure frequencies of common events of interest by time, place and person • Identify possible risk factors • Test hypotheses	• As above	• As above
	Case (series) report	Describe one case (or small number of cases) with an unusual attribute, related possibly to a single cause		• Report interesting or unusual cases • Identify their common attributes	• Cheap, quick and easy to conduct	• Small numbers • No control group and cases may be unrepresentative

Table 2.3 (Continued)

Type	Subtype	Graphical representation	Objectives	Advantages	Disadvantages
	Ecological studies (aggregate or descriptive study)	For aggregate unit(s), usually defined geographically, compare frequencies in exposures and outcomes between groups (ecologic comparison study; see diagram) or over time (ecologic trend study)	• Generate hypotheses	• Cheap and quick (use routinely collected data) • Can generate hypotheses to test at the individual level • Appropriate if the exposure is geographic; varies much more between than within populations; or is less prone to measurement error at the group level than individual level	• Design is incomplete: do not know the number of exposed cases • Does not permit causal inferences • Conclusions may be spurious when observations about a group are applied uncritically to individuals • Routine data may not adequately measure the factors of interest

Graphical representation diagram:

N_1 — E
N_1 — $\tilde{E}$ / C
$\hat{C}$ / E

N_2 — $\tilde{E}$ / C
$\hat{C}$

Table 2.4. Cases Study Designs

	Single case designs	Multiple case designs
Holistic case (single unit of analysis)	Type 1	Type 2
Embedded case (multiple units of analysis, i.e. the case is disaggregated)	Type 3	Type 4

CHOOSING STUDY DESIGNS

How can we decide which quantitative study design(s) to use? We could refer to the hierarchies that rank them in order of decreasing internal validity. These are intended to grade the ability of different study designs to minimize bias and produce the best 'evidence' capable of answering particular types of questions. Most of the hierarchies relate to the capacity of studies to deliver evidence of effectiveness but evidence hierarchies have also been developed to answer questions about areas such as etiology, diagnosis and prognosis [16]. Systematic reviews are commonly reported to yield the highest level of evidence for all study questions. However, for undertaking original research the ideal design is usually stated to be, for example, a randomized trial to answer questions about interventions, and a cohort study for questions about prognosis and diagnosis [16].

Evidence hierarchies have not gone uncontested. Criticisms of, and alternatives to, them [17-19] have been suggested for a variety of reasons including:

1. In practice, factors besides the research question can influence the choice of study design. These include ethical considerations, what is feasible, and the relevancy of the results to the context in which they will be used. So, experimentation is sometimes, for example, unethical (Table 7.1). More generally it may be 'unnecessary,' 'inappropriate,' 'impossible' or 'inadequate' (Table 7.2) [20]. Unlike observational studies it also provides evidence shorn of context. This characteristic, along with issues such as the artificiality of randomized trials, suggests that: 'the notion that information from randomised trials represents a gold standard while that derived from observational studies is viewed as wrong, may be too simplistic. An alternative perspective is that randomized trials provide an indication of the minimum effect of an intervention whereas observational studies offer an estimate of the maximum effect' [20, p. 1218].

2. The ideal study design is not necessarily the only or most appropriate criterion for what constitutes 'best evidence.' Evidence hierarchies fail to acknowledge that different forms of evidence vary in kind and not merely in degree. Study designs (e.g. randomized trials and qualitative research) can also be complementary rather than necessarily alternatives [18].

3. There are competing hierarchies of research evidence for effectiveness [21]. A new system (GRADE) of grading the level of research evidence and the strength of recommendations is intended to be applicable across different health care interventions and contexts [22]. However, why this system is the right or only one is unclear.

4. The epistemic superiority of randomized trials over well-conducted observational studies of interventions has been challenged [23-25]. The argument goes that the latter studies do not overestimate effects of the intervention compared with randomized trials on the same topic.

MEASURES OF FREQUENCY

For each study design, we can produce and use measures of frequency and measures of effect. To understand the most commonly used measures of frequency, it helps to distinguish between the concepts of *incidence* and *prevalence*. Figure 2.2 aims to support this need. It shows that the incidence of a given condition or characteristic is the number of new cases of this condition which develop during a specified time period in the population. Incidence measures require longitudinal data, for example from experiments, cohort studies or disease registers.

In contrast the prevalence of a condition is shown to refer to the proportion of the population that has the condition at a designated time. It is a measure of the frequency of all (new and existing) cases, and so describes the probability of cases occurring and the burden on the population. Assessments of prevalences are common, for example, in descriptive epidemiological studies. The prevalence of a condition is proportional to the incidence times the duration of the condition.

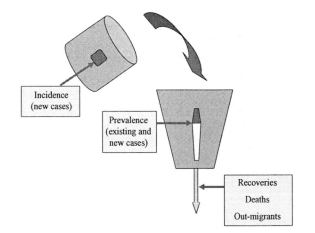

Figure 2.2. Comparing the Concepts of Incidence and Prevalence.

Consider four measures of frequency:

1. A *count* is the number of times that a particular event occurs in a set time period. Counts are usually expressed relative to the size of the group at risk but for some conditions (e.g. human-human transmission of bird flu), even a single suspected case would be of health significance.
2. A *ratio* (*a* / *b*) compares two numbers in groups that can be mutually exclusive; for example a patient: doctor ratio of 2000: 1 or a sex ratio at birth of 105 (105 boys to every 100 girls).

3. A *proportion* (*a / (a + b)*) is the ratio of a part to a whole; the numerator is always part of the denominator. A proportion may be expressed as a decimal fraction in the range of 0 to 1 (e.g. 0.1); as a vulgar fraction (e.g. 1/10th); or as a percentage (e.g. 10%). Proportions tell us what fraction of the population is affected by the condition of interest. Some proportions are misidentified as rates (e.g. the case fatality rate). Examples of different types of proportions, associated with the different study designs, include cumulative incidences (intervention studies and cohort studies) and prevalences (cross-sectional studies).

4. A *rate* (*Δa / Δb*, i.e. the change in *a*, per unit change in *b*) reports the number of new outcome events (numerator) per unit of population per unit of time (denominator). The denominator can be represented as the sum of the time at risk by all study individuals during the observation period. In measuring how quickly the event of interest is occurring, a rate can range from 0 to infinity. The calculation of rates requires data to reflect change in the population over time. Therefore the crude death rate, for example, is a 'true rate' because the numerator typically comes from a register of deaths and each person in the population is assumed to contribute one year of follow-up. In contrast, prevalences are not rates because they can be expressed only in relation to the population at a fixed 'point' in time (which can stretch to become a period of time). An *index* is an example of a *pseudo-rate* because the true denominator (population at risk) is unknown, requiring the use of a related denominator.

Figure 2.3 reinforces how to determine whether measures of frequency are ratios, proportions or rates. Table 2.5 builds on this discussion by describing and evaluating different types of proportions and rates respectively. We will then elaborate on standardized rates, using worked examples in Tables 2.6 and 2.7 to show how to standardize rates directly and indirectly.

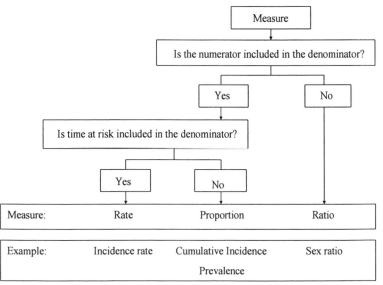

Figure 2.3. Measures of Frequency.
Reprinted (with small changes) from The Lancet, Vol. 359, Grimes DA, Schulz KF, An overview of clinical research: the lay of the land, 57-61, Copyright 5 January 2002, with permission from Elsevier.

Table 2.5. Types of Proportions and Rates

Type	Example	Equation for the example given	Advantages	Disadvantages
Proportions				
Incidence risks (cumulative incidence)	Risk of cancer over a specified time period such as 10 years	$$\frac{\text{New cancer diagnoses in specified time period}}{\text{Population at risk of developing the cancer during the same period}} * 100{,}000$$	• Estimate the (conditional) probability that all members of the population who are free of the disease (or event) at the study outset, but are at risk of it occurring, will develop it during the study period. Can be used, for example, for surveillance purposes	• Assume that people have equal exposure yet they may differ in their period of exposure. Therefore, these measures are not true rates because the person-time at risk is unknown
Point prevalences (and period prevalences – including lifetime prevalences)	Cancer point prevalence (and cancer period prevalence)	$$\frac{\text{All cases of cancer (old and new) at a fixed point in time (or alternatively during a specified period of time)}}{\text{Population at risk at that time}} * 100{,}000$$	• Reveal the burden of the health problem at a fixed point in time or during a specified period • Reveal population requirements for health care resources	• As above for incidences • Differences in prevalence may be due to population changes rather than incidence
Rates				
Incidence rates (Incidence densities)	Cancer incidence per 100,000 person-years	$$\frac{\text{New cancer diagnoses in specified time period}}{\text{Sum of person-years at risk}} * 100{,}000$$ To see how to calculate person-years at risk, consider the example of 500 person-years of observation. This may represent 500 people each observed for one year; 50 people each observed for 10 years; or, when people are followed for variable lengths of time, some combination such as 40 people each observed for 5 years and 50 people each observed for 6 years	• Apply to 'cases' or, in certain recurrent diseases such as asthma, to events or episodes • Take into account the size of the population at risk and the duration of observation for each individual • Are dynamic, not static • Can be used to help investigate the causes of health problems and the effectiveness of interventions	• Cannot reveal precisely when the case or event occurs • The rate at which it develops over time is not necessarily constant

Table 2.5 (Continued)

Type	Example	Equation for the example given	Advantages	Disadvantages
Crude rates	Crude death rate	$\dfrac{\text{Deaths in calendar year}}{\text{Population at mid-year}} * 1000$	• Are easy and quick to compute and readily understood	• Take no account of the population composition (e.g. age and sex structure)
Rates *specific* for factors such as age and sex	Age-sex specific death rates	$\dfrac{\text{Deaths in calendar year to men (or women) in each specified age group}}{\text{Mid-year population for the same age-sex group}} * 1000$	• Are an absolute measure and a useful tool for comparison	• Not one number, making comparisons difficult and tedious
Synthetic rates	Total fertility rate	$\dfrac{\text{Sum of 5-year age-specific fertility rates (ASFRs) per 1000}}{1000} * 5$ Interpretation: number of children born to an imaginary woman if she survived her reproductive years and experienced the ASFRs in the year in question	• Provide a single figure measure, e.g. of fertility independent of age structure	• Require a lot of data • Not easily interpreted • Can be greatly distorted by shifts in the timing of childbearing

Table 2.5 (Continued)

Type	Example	Equation for the example given	Advantages	Disadvantages
Cohort rates [26]	Cohort fertility rate (CFR)	$\dfrac{\text{Sum of ASFRs for each birth cohort}}{1000} * 5$ Interpretation: average number of children born by age 50 to women in a named birth cohort	• Considers the experience of a single group over time • Can explain levels and trends	• Require long and consistent time series of data • Introduce the problem of 'censoring' (experience of recent cohorts is unknown)

ASFRs: New Zealand, 1975-2005

Age group	1975	1980	1985	1990	1995	2000	2005
15-19	55	38	30	35	33	28	27
20-24	158	127	104	103	83	78	69
25-29	157	147	145	149	123	113	107
30-34	70	68	79	107	106	113	120
35-39	25	21	22	37	44	53	64
40-44	7	4	4	5	7	10	12
45-49	1	0	0	0	0	0	1

$$\text{CFR for 1955-9 cohort} = \frac{55 + 127 + 145 + 107 + 44 + 10 + 1}{1000} * 5 = 2.4$$

Table 2.5 (Continued)

Type	Example	Equation for the example given	Advantages	Disadvantages
Rates standardized or adjusted for differences in factors such as age	Age-standardized death rates	Two approaches: Direct standardization Indirect standardization	• Adjust for effects of age structure (and/or other factors) in order to compare rates between populations in different areas or over time	• Are fictitious • Indicate poorly the absolute level (e.g. of mortality) in a population
Change rates		$$\frac{\text{New value} - \text{old value}}{\text{Old value}} * 100$$		

Standardized Rates

Comparisons of rates across different populations are not always straightforward. One difficulty is variations, between populations, in factors that influence the variable of interest but are not the real focus of attention. Adjustment seeks to remove the effects of such extraneous factors that distort or *confound* comparisons (see Figure 6.2). One form of adjustment is standardization [27].

A *standardized rate* is a rate that uses weighted averages to adjust for differences (e.g. in age structure) between populations. Standardization permits valid comparisons in event occurrence between populations, for example at different points in time, in different geographic areas or in different groups such as ethnic groups. Standardization can be direct or indirect.

Direct standardization, for example by age, calculates a weighted average of a population's age-specific rates. The weights are the population in the equivalent age group of the standard (or reference) population. Table 2.6 illustrates how to standardize death rates directly by age. It shows what the mortality in New Zealand would have been in 2004 if the population age structure had been the same as in 1986. Note that the age-standardized death rate in 2004 is less than the crude death rate for 2004, and the lower crude death rate in 2004 than in 1986 underestimates the size of the reduction in mortality over time. Standardization has therefore removed the tendency of population aging to dilute the reduction in death rates between 1986 and 2004. Since the 1986 population was our standard, the standardized rate in 1986 is the same as the crude rate for that year.

Table 2.6. Direct Standardization of New Zealand Death Rates, 1986 And 2004, by Age

Age	Standard population December 1986	Population, December 1986		Population, December 2004	
		Age-specific death rates per 1000	Expected deaths (2) * (3)	Age-specific death rates per 1000	Expected deaths (2) * (5)
(1)	(2)	(3)	(4)	(5)	(6)
0-14	793,490	1.1	873	0.5	397
15-64	2,139,600	3.3	7061	2.1	4493
65+	343,830	55.5	19083	45.6	15,679
Total	3,276,920		27017		20569
Standardized death rate per 1000		8.2 ((4)/(2)) * 1000		6.3 ((5)/(2)) *1000	
Crude death rate (CDR)		8.3		7.2	

Indirect standardization applies category-specific reference rates to the population in the equivalent category of the study group. Table 2.7 shows how to age-standardize indirectly. It shows what the mortality in 2004 would have been in New Zealand if the death rates by age had been the same as in 1986. Mortality in 2004 is below expectation, reducing the crude death rate in 2004 by almost 1 death per 1000. Because directly standardized rates are based on the same set of weights (the age distribution of the standard population), they can be validly compared in relative or absolute terms. In contrast, since indirectly standardized rates are based on each study population's own age distribution, the standardized rates for several study populations cannot be validly compared (unless they have similar age distributions) [28]; the only valid comparison is between the study population and the reference population because of the use of weights from the study population. However, when stratum-specific numbers are small, direct standardization is the less robust approach; and indirect standardization avoids the distortions that unstable rates produce with direct standardization.

Table 2.7. Indirect Standardization of New Zealand Death Rates, 1986 and 2004, by Age

Age	December 1986 death rates per 1000	December 1986 Population	Expected deaths (2) * (3)	December 2004 Population	Expected deaths (2) * (5)
(1)	(2)	(3)	(4)	(5)	(6)
0-14	1.1	793,490	873	884,660	973
15-64	3.3	2,139,600	7061	2,691,920	8883
65+	55.5	343,830	19083	485,860	26,965
Total		3,276,920	27,017	4,062,440	36,821
Total deaths registered (actual deaths)			27,045		28,419
Standardized Mortality Ratio (SMR) = (actual deaths / expected deaths)			1.0		0.77
Indirect standardized rate per 1000 = (SMR * CDR of standard population			8.3		6.4

Measures of Effect

Besides measures of frequency, we are likely to encounter measures of effect. The latter measures express the risk or probability of an association between particular exposures and outcomes of interest. This probability is usually applied to non-recurrent events, or first episodes. Table 2.8 shows how to calculate absolute and relative measures of effect when our data are summarized in a 2 * 2 table (study participants did or did not have the outcome in the presence of absence of a specified exposure) from studies with count denominators and person-time denominators respectively.

All the measures apply to intervention studies [29] and cohort studies [30]. Only some of the measures apply to case-control [30 31] and cross-sectional studies [32].

Table 2.8. Measuring the Risks of Benefit or Harm From Exposure/Treatment

		Outcome event			Person-time *(PT)*
		Present	Absent		
Exposure/treatment	Present	*a*	*b*	*e (a + b)*	$PT_{Exposed}$
	Absent	*c*	*d*	*f (c + d)*	$PT_{Unexposed}$
		g (a + c)	*h (b + d)*	*i*	PT_{Total}

Measure	Description	Equation
Absolute risk		
• Experimental event rate (EER) or proportion of the exposed experiencing the outcome of interest	Actual risk or probability of the event occurring in the presence of exposure	a / e
• Controlled event rate (CER) or proportion of the unexposed experiencing the outcome of interest	Actual risk or probability of the event occurring in the absence of exposure	c / f
Risk ratio (relative risk, RR)	Ratio of two absolute risks. It measures the effect of an exposure on risk. A beneficial effect produces a RR < 1. Subtracting this number from 1 gives the Relative Risk Reduction. A harmful exposure yields a RR > 1. Examples of the RR are the cumulative incidence RR and the prevalence RR	$(a / e) / (c / f)$ (or EER / CER)
Rate ratio	Ratio of two incidence rates	For incidence rates: $(a / PT_{Exposed}) / (c / PT_{Unexposed})$
Relative risk reduction or relative risk increase	Change in the relative risk. Large relative risk reductions can appear impressive. However, the same relative risk reduction can conceal different changes in absolute risk, and so is not very useful in everyday clinical practice	$(a / e) - (c / f)) / (c / f)$ (or (EER – CER) / CER)
Risk difference (attributable risk or absolute risk reduction, ARR)	Difference in absolute risk attributable to some exposure	(EER) – (CER)
Rate difference	Difference between two incidence rates	$(a / PT_{Exposed}) - (c / PT_{Unexposed})$
Odds ratio (OR)	A ratio of the odds (number of present events divided by the number of absent events) in the exposed group relative to the non-exposed group. Appropriate to case-control studies, where it is an estimate of the relative risk	$(a / b) / (c / d) = a * d / c * b$
Number needed to treat (NNT)	Number of patients it is necessary to treat to prevent one adverse event. The best NNT is 1. Higher NNTs are less good. NNTs can be used to compare similar treatments	1 / ARR

Table 2.8 (Continued)

Measure	Description	Equation
Attributable risk for the exposed(often expressed as a percentage)	Proportion of all exposed cases attributable to the exposure	(EER – CER) / EER This is equivalent to: (RR – 1)/ RR, and in case-control studies: (OR -1) / OR
Population attributable risk	Proportion of all cases (exposed and unexposed) attributable to the exposure	p (RR – 1) / (p (RR – 1) + 1) where p = proportion of total population that is exposed

SCREENING AND DIAGNOSTIC TESTING

Other measures of effect relate to screening and diagnostic testing. The Standards for Reporting Diagnostic Accuracy (STARD) statement helps to assess the validity of studies that use these measures to evaluate the accuracy of screening and diagnostic tests [33]. These studies have traditionally compared test results against a reference ('gold') standard by focusing on the sensitivity and specificity of the test (and its positive and negative predictive values) (see Table 2.9).

Table 2.9. Accuracy of Screening and Diagnostic Testing for Groups

Test Result (or symptoms)	Condition Present	Condition Absent	Total
Positive	a True positive	b False positive	$a + b$
Negative	c False negative	d True negative	$c + d$
Total	$a + c$	$b + d$	$a + c + b + d$

Test sensitivity = $a / (a + c)$
Test specificity = $d / (b + d)$
Test positive predictive value = $a / (a + b)$
Test negative predictive value = $d / (c + d)$
Diagnostic accuracy = $(a + d) / (a + b + c + d)$.

These measures of population risk do not translate easily to individuals. However, the process needed to do this is intuitively familiar. For example, have you asked someone how they are today? If so, you have performed a diagnostic test! The same process can be formalized to estimate the probability that an individual or group has some target condition of interest. Specifically, it is necessary first to estimate the *pre-test probability* of the condition. From this measure and the *likelihood ratio,* the *post-test probability* can be calculated. Table 2.10 considers these measures.

Table 2.10. Screening and Diagnostic Testing for Individuals and Groups

	Definition	Source	Hazards or benefits
Pre-test probability (prior probability or prevalence)	Probability of having the condition *before* doing the test; i.e., the proportion of people with the condition in the population at risk at a specific time or in a specified time interval	Experience and literature From Table 2.9: $(a + c) / (a + b + c + d)$	Pretest probability can help in: • Deciding whether to test • Selecting one or more diagnostic tests • Interpreting the test results • Deciding whether to start treatment However, a low pre-test probability produces a high risk of a *false positive* result. A high pre-test probability produces a high risk of a *false negative* result
Likelihood ratio	Likelihood of having the condition A *positive likelihood ratio* is the likelihood of having the condition given a positive test result A *negative likelihood ratio* is the likelihood of having the condition given a negative test result	Literature Likelihood ratio for a positive test (LR+) = True positive rate / False positive rate $= \dfrac{a / (a + c)}{b / (b + d)}$ = sensitivity (1 – specificity) Likelihood ratio for a negative test (LR-) = FN rate /TN rate $= \dfrac{c / (a + c)}{d / (b + d)}$ = (1 – sensitivity) / specificity	Time is required to search the literature Reported test properties may or may not be applicable to your own patients [34] However, likelihood ratios: • Have an intuitive meaning • Emphasize that the diagnosis is never certain • Are independent of the condition prevalence • Permit quantification of the probability that an individual or group has the condition of interest

Table 2.10 (Continued)

	Definition	Source	Hazards or benefits
Post-test probability	Probability of having the condition *after* knowing the test result; i.e. the proportion of people with a particular test result who have the condition of interest	Bayes theorem tells us that the pre-test *odds* of having the condition, multiplied by the likelihood ratio, yields the post-test *odds* of having the condition (odds = probability (p) / ($1-p$)). Easier to use, however, is Bayes nomogram (see below):	The post-test probability provides a post-test quantitative estimate of the probability of the condition being present in an individual or group. It avoids, therefore, the 'one size fits all' approach (for which guidelines have been criticized). But it reflects statistical uncertainty around estimates of both the pre-test probability and test performance

Positive likelihood ratio ———
Negative likelihood ratio ——

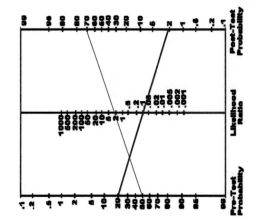

ADDITIONAL STATISTICAL CONCEPTS

To prepare for subsequent chapters, we need to look at two statistical concepts relevant to measures of sample estimates. These are 'p values' and confidence limits. Both concepts are part of inferential (or inductive) statistics, which aims to infer whether patterns in a probability sample are representative of the population from which the sample was selected.

P-Values

The main methods used in inferential statistics are hypothesis testing and estimation. A *(null) hypothesis* about a population characteristic (parameter) is put forward and a test is performed to assess whether the data are *strong* enough to reject it. In testing the hypothesis, a p value, understood most simply, is the probability 'that any particular outcome would have arisen by chance' [35]. More accurately it is the probability of getting a result at least as extreme as the one observed if the (null) hypothesis (e.g. no difference (on what is being compared) between the groups) is true. This probability is assumed to be a random variable (come from a recognizable probability distribution), which varies from sample to sample. So, we cannot compare p values across different samples, tests or experiments.

It is typical to reject the null hypothesis if the p value is less than or equal to the *'significance level'* (also called the rejection level, which is typically 0.05 or 0.01) that has been fixed before examining the data. Usually represented by the Greek letter α (alpha), the significance level is also the (pretest) probability of rejecting the null hypothesis when it is true (a Type I error, or false positive).

It is important to balance the risk of this error against the risk of not rejecting the null hypothesis when we should reject it (a Type 2 error, or false negative, designated by the Greek letter β (beta)). This error can occur when, for example, the rejection level is set too low, given the study power (($1-\beta$) or probability that the null hypothesis will be rejected if it is not true).

It is best to report actual p values, for example because the smaller the p value below the significance level, the stronger is the rejection of the null hypothesis. However, it is commonplace to see $p < 0.05$ ($p < 5\%$) or $p < 0.01$ ($p < 1\%$), in part because p values are often approximations.

Non-statistically significant findings indicate an absence of evidence of differences rather than no difference; the result could reflect too few participants or our particular sample. So, quantitative results may be statistically significant but not clinically important. Also, p values say nothing about the size of the effects that may lead to us to reject or fail to reject the null hypothesis.

Confidence Intervals

These are 'margins of error' around sample estimates, which take a range of values (estimated from sample data) that have a selected likelihood of including the unknown population parameter. For example, 95% confidence intervals tell us that if, hypothetically, repeated, independent samples were taken from the same population, in 95% of the samples the true value of the estimates (whose distribution is assumed to be 'normal') would lay between the lower and upper confidence limits.

Confidence intervals therefore indicate the *precision* of sample estimates, and range of possible effect *sizes*. They also avoid confusion over the term 'significant;' remind us that all estimates are subject to error; and contain information about the *p* value. The latter can be inferred, for example, from whether a finding of 'no difference' falls within the confidence interval, if we are 'expressing the result as a dichotomy (that is, is the hypothesis "proved" or "disproved"?)' [35]. Thus, a 95% confidence interval (e.g. around the difference between means) that does not include 0 (no difference) is statistically significant at the 5% level; if the confidence interval includes 0, the effect may or may not be statistically significant at the 5% level. Similarly, if two 95% confidence intervals do not overlap, we can infer that the difference between them is statistically significant at the 5% level. If they do overlap, the difference may be statistically significant at the 5% level.

Confidence intervals are calculated from the standard error (SE) of the parameter estimate. The SE is the standard deviation (a measure of the spread or dispersion) of the distribution of an infinite number of hypothetical repeated samples. A SE of 0 indicates no random error. In general, the larger the sample size, the smaller the SE – and the narrower the confidence interval.

REFERENCES

[1]   Demeterio FI. Logic, the philosophy of systematic thinking and argumentation. *Diwatao* 2001;1(1). http://www.geocities.com/philodept/diwatao/logic.htm

[2]   Cresswell J. *Research design: Qualitative, quantitative and mixed methods approaches.* 2nd Edition. Thousand Oaks, CA: Sage, 2003.

[3]   Jackson R, Ameratunga S, Broad J, Connor J, Lethaby A, Robb G, et al. The Gate frame: critical appraisal with pictures. *Evidence-Based Med* 200;11:35-38.

[4]   Popper K. *The Logic of Scientific Discovery.* New York: NY Basic Books 1959.

[5]   Des Jarlais DC, Lyles C, Crepaz N. Improving the reporting quality of nonrandomized evaluations of behavioral and public health interventions: The TREND statement. *Am. J. Pub. Health* 2004;94:361-6.

[6]   Harris A, McGregor J, Perencevich E, Furuno J, Zhu J, DE P, et al. The use and interpretation of quasi-experimental studies in medical informatics. *J. Am. Med. Inform. Assoc.* 2006;13:16-23.

[7]   Eccles M, Grimshaw J, Campbell M, Ramsay C. Research designs for studies evaluating the effectiveness of change and improvement strategies. *Qual. Saf. Health Care* 2003;12:47-52.

[8]   Kleinbaum DG, Kupper LL, Morgenstern H. *Epidemiologic Research. Principles and Quantitative Methods.* London: Lifetime Learning Publications, 1982.

[9]   Ragin C, Becker H. *What is a case? Exploring the Foundations of Social Inquiry.* Cambridge, UK: Cambridge University Press, 1992.

[10]   Yin R. *Case Study Research: Design and Methods. Applied Social Research Methods Series.* 3rd Edition. Thousand Oaks, California: Sage, 2002.

[11] Bergen A. A case for case studies: exploring the use of case study design in community nursing research. *J. Adv. Nurs.* 2000;31:926-34.

[12] Stake R. Qualitative case studies. In: Denzin N, Lincoln Y (eds). *The Sage Handbook of Qualitative Research.* 3rd Edition. London: Thousand Oaks, 2005:443-66.

[13] Lijphart A. Comparative politics and the comparative method. *Am. Pol. Sci. Rev.* 1971;65:682-93.

[14] Jensen J, Rodgers R. Cumulating the intellectual gold of case study research. *Pub. Admin. Rev.* 2001;61:236-46.

[15] Neuman W. *Social Research Methods. Qualitative and Quantitative Approaches.* 5th Edition. London: Allyn and Bacon, 2003.

[16] Phillips P, Ball C, Sackett D, Badenoch D, Straus S, Haynes B, et al. *Levels of Evidence and Grades of Recommendation.* Oxford: Oxford Centre for Evidence-Based Medicine, 2001.

[17] Rychetnik L, Frommer M, Hawe P, Shiell A. Criteria for evaluating evidence on public health interventions. *J. Epidemiol. Community Health* 2002;56:119-27.

[18] Pettigrew M, Roberts H. Evidence, hierarchies, and typologies: horses for courses. *J Epidemiol Community Health* 2003;57:527-9.

[19] Evans D. Hierarchy of evidence: a framework for ranking evidence evaluating healthcare interventions. *J. Clin. Nursing.* 2003;12:77-84.

[20] Black N. Why we need observational studies to evaluate the effectiveness of health care. *BMJ* 1996;312:1215-8.

[21] Upshur R. Are all evidence based practices alike? Problems in the ranking of evidence. *Can. Med. Assoc. J.* 2003;169:672-3.

[22] Grades of Recommendation A, Development and Evaluation (GRADE) Working Group,. Grading quality of evidence and strength of recommendations. *BMJ* 2004;328:1490-4.

[23] Benson K, Hartz A. A comparison of observational studies and randomised controlled trials. *N. Eng. J. Med.* 2000;342:1878-86.

[24] Concato J, Shah N, Horowitz R. Randomised controlled trials, observational studies, and the hierarchy of research designs. *N. Eng. J. Med* .2000;342:1887-92.

[25] Worrall J. What evidence in evidence-based medicine? *Philos Sci* 2002;69:S316-S330.

[26] Newell C. *Methods and Models in Demography.* London: Belhaven Press, 1988.

[27] Pollard A, Yusuf F, Pollard G. *Demographic techniques* 3rd Edition. Sydney: AS Wilson, 1995.

[28] Rixom A. Performance league tables. Use of indirect standardisation is inappropriate. *BMJ* 2002;325:177-8.

[29] O'Connell R, Gebski V, AC K. Making sense of trial results: outcomes and estimation. *Med. J. Aust.* 2004;180:128-30.

[30] Rockett I. Population and health: An introduction to epidemiology. *Pop. Bull.* 1999;54:1-46.

[31] Schlesselman JJ. *Case-control Studies.* New York: Oxford University Press, 1982.

[32] World Health Organization (WHO) Regional Office for the Western Pacific. *Health Research Methodology.* Manila: WHO, 1992.

[33] Bossuyt P, Reitsma J, Bruns D, Gatsonis C, Glasziou P, Irwig L, et al. The STARD Statement for Reporting Studies of Diagnostic Accuracy: Explanation and Elaboration. *Ann. Intern. Med* .2003;138:W1-W12.

[34] Jaeschke R, Gordon H, Guyatt G, Sackett D. Users' guides to the medical literature. III. How to use an article about a diagnostic test. B. what are the results and will they help me in caring for my patients? *JAMA* 1994;271:703-7.

[35] Greenhalgh, T. Statistics for the non-statistician. II: "Significant" relations and their pitfalls. *BMJ* 1997; 315: 422-5.

Chapter 3

LITERATURE REVIEWS

OBJECTIVES

By the time you have completed this chapter, you should be able to:

1. Describe different types and sources of literature relevant to your research question
2. Describe the need for, and compare types of, literature reviews
3. Conduct a systematic review
4. Discuss approaches to evidence synthesis
5. Understand how to produce a meta-analysis
6. Critique an existing systematic review or meta-analysis

PREVIEW

Literature reviews synthesize evidence from different sources in order to keep efficiently up to date with, and make effective use of, past and new research developments. For example, formulating a good research question, and linking past research to future study, depends on the prior identification, retrieval and review of the evidence already produced and reported in the literature. This chapter considers how to search the literature and produce different types of literature review. It also considers different approaches to the synthesis of quantitative and qualitative evidence.

TYPES OF LITERATURE

In general, we can distinguish between two types of literature: the published literature and the so-called 'grey' literature. Table 3.1 compares these broad types.

Table 3.1. Types of Literature

	Description	Types	Key sources
Published literature	Literature published commercially	• Books • Journal articles	• Library catalogues • Electronic databases such as CENTRAL (Cochrane Central Register of controlled trials), MEDLINE/PubMed, EMBASE, Current Contents and CINAHL • Academic and professional journals • Reference lists of published articles Personal communication
Grey literature	Non-conventional literature, semi- or not commercially published	• Theses and dissertations • Meeting and conference proceedings • Newsletters • Reports, including government publications • Electronic networks • Brochures and pamphlets	Library databases: • Digital dissertations • Networked Digital Library of Theses • Conference Papers Index Internet databases: • HTA Database • SIGLE (subscription only) • The Grey Journal (TGJ) is a flagship journal for the grey literature Personal communication

LITERATURE REVIEWS

1. Rationale

The explosion in the volume of research means that no health professional can read even a modest proportion of what has been produced. Readers may not have the time and skills to appraise research. Even when these resources are available, individual studies are seldom sufficient in themselves. They sometimes conflict and may, for example, lack statistical power, be context-dependent, reflect researcher bias, lack evidence of reproducibility from other theoretical and methodological perspectives, and not explain why and when interventions work or not [1].

There is pressure nevertheless to know what the best available evidence is, and to inform timely decision-making. By bringing evidence together from different sources, reviews of the literature can help to meet these needs. The reviews can summarize and synthesize what has been written on a topic and reveal what appears not to be known. They can thereby support, and highlight opportunities for, the use and generation of knowledge in policy development, specific management contexts, clinical practice and future research.

2. Types

Table 3.2 compares and evaluates three different types of literature review that we may find or produce: the narrative review, the realist review and the systematic review.

3. Methodology for Systematic Reviews

Table 3.3 elaborates on how to produce a systematic review. It summarizes the different steps involved in planning the review, executing the plan and then reporting and disseminating the results.

As noted in Table 3.3, a key step in conducting a systematic review is data synthesis. We will elaborate on this issue in the next section of this Chapter. However, first, Table 3.4 will look at how to assess the degree and impact of heterogeneity between study findings, since the results of this assessment will influence how we choose to synthesize the data collected from individual studies.

EVIDENCE SYNTHESIS

Evidence (or data) synthesis is a key stage of a literature review (see Table 3.3). Indeed, it is so important that we will consider it now in detail. Evidence synthesis aims to juxtapose and/or integrate the research evidence (the grounds for believing or claiming something) available from different primary studies. It can (1) be an additive process of accumulating knowledge on a given topic, (2) refute or resolve arguments or (3) play an interpretative role by facilitating reconceptualization across studies [7]. Deliberative processes can be used to combine different forms of evidence [8]. Using a similar structure to the discussion of different types of literature review (Table 3.2), the following section will discuss different types of evidence synthesis [9], drawing on the approaches described in Table 3.5.

Meta-Analysis

Meta-analysis is an approach associated with quantitative synthesis in systematic reviews (Table 3.5). It refers to statistical analysis and, if appropriate, to statistical pooling of the summary results of all relevant prior studies – i.e. since 'meta' means 'about' (or 'behind' or of a 'higher order') a meta-analysis is strictly an analysis of analyses. Table 3.6 provides an overview of characteristics of this approach. Table 3.7 elaborates on the production of pooled estimates of effect size.

Table 3.2. Types of Literature Review

Type of review	Description	Purpose	Method	Advantages	Disadvantages
Narrative review (also known as a comprehensive review or an integrative review) [2]	Overview of evidence addressing a research question	Summarize the evidence and identify gaps	Idiosyncratic, iterative, often informal and subjective	• Relatively easy and quick to produce. • Can accommodate diverse methodologies, types of data and cutting edge developments that may continue to evolve after the review starts	• Subjective and unscientific; prone to bias and error. • Practical difficulties: can be unmanageable
Systematic review	Group of similar studies summarized through a systematic and comprehensive review	Objectively answer a focused research question, e.g. on whether something 'works'. Help to limit error, resolve uncertainty and keep up with the research evidence	Systematically identify, scrutinize, tabulate and integrate all the relevant studies	• Explicit, detailed and transparent • Minimizes bias and random error • Yields reliable and reproducible results applicable across settings and populations	• Need clear rules for producing a review before starting it • Can be too restrictive • May lack validity because of the poor quality of component trials and reporting biases
Realist review [1 3]	A kind of systematic review suited to complex social interventions	Increase understanding of how something works (or not), under what conditions, and with what effect	'Realist' approach to evaluation. Interprets empirical evidence through the lens of theory	• Eclectic and flexible. Refines theory. • Involves and influences end-users	• May lack feasibility. Similar limitations to qualitative research; e.g. requires reflexivity and an audit trail

Table 3.3. Steps in Conducting a Systematic Review [4 5]

1. Plan the review: Specify the purpose of the review Establish a need for the review Prepare a proposal and review protocol	• Identify potentially relevant questions, which are amenable to review • Find and appraise any relevant, existing reviews in order to establish the scope of, and need for, a new review • Document the methodology for a literature review to answer a clearly focused question, and report and disseminate its findings
2. Do the review: Define study eligibility criteria (inclusion and exclusion criteria) Produce a search strategy and comprehensively search the literature	• Define eligible participants, settings, interventions, comparisons, outcomes and other study attributes (e.g. study designs, languages of reporting, period of coverage, and requirements for methodological quality) • Define search terms that appear to meet the eligibility criteria and apply thoroughly to the key data sources • Hand search journals as an adjunct to searching electronic databases. • Check the reference lists of retrieved works; other reviews; and, for early searches, the print versions of electronic databases
Select studies to include	• Review study abstracts (where available) and, if necessary, retrieve the full text of all studies identified through application of the search strategy • Use independent, possibly blinded reviewers to apply all the eligibility (inclusion and exclusion) criteria specified in the review protocol; check the study eligibility; and resolve disagreements using decision rules set at the outset. Record the excluded studies with reasons for their exclusion • Include grey literature to minimize the risk of publication bias. Compared with unpublished randomized trials, published randomized trials are generally larger and may show an overall greater treatment effect. Including unpublished trials may minimize the risk of introducing bias into reviews. However, published trials may be of higher quality than unpublished trials [6] • Assess each study's methodological quality. Use it as an eligibility criterion or for other purposes, such as to help explain differences in results between studies
Assemble dataset	• Design, pilot test and, if necessary, revise a standardized data extraction form (e.g. http://www.york.ac.uk/inst/crd/pdf/crd4_app3.pdf) with clear decision rules • Involve independent reviewers in data extraction, data recording and checking the reliability of these processes • If necessary, seek to collect missing information from the original investigators

Table 3.3 (Continued)

Synthesize data

- Tabulate characteristics of each included study to permit comparisons (on variables such as year, settings, patients, intervention, comparison, outcome and quality)
  - Graph and examine results from the individual trials to:
    a. Aid a descriptive synthesis of the results
    b. Look for heterogeneity between study findings. This refers to the presence of greater variability in effect size estimates than is expected from sampling error alone – or, put simply, the results of the individual studies differ strongly, producing 'strange fruit' (as in the title of the song, 'Strange fruit,' made famous by Billie Holiday).

Some heterogeneity is unavoidable in systematic reviews, but it is important to assess whether its degree and impact (Table 3.4 and Figure 3.2) undermine quantitative synthesis of the data from the individual studies (Tables 3.5-3.6) to produce a single pooled estimate of effect size (the strength of relationship between an exposure and an outcome)

  c. Decide whether to include a meta-analysis (Table 3.6) of all or some trials in order to estimate a pooled effect
  d. Check the robustness of the review findings against different underlying assumptions. As part of a sensitivity analysis (which explores 'what ifs' associated with changes to the data and methods), check whether the studies are biased toward reporting results that:
     - are statistically significant (publication bias),
     - are published in English (language bias),
     - are published more than once (multiple publication bias)
     - are cited frequently (citation bias),
     - report dramatic results, disproportionately in small studies (small study bias)
  e. Look for asymmetry in 'funnel plots,' which can reveal bias (Figure 3.1). These scatter plots typically display, for each included study, (a) the effect size (horizontal axis) versus (b) a measure of the study size (vertical axis). Precision in estimating the effect size increases as the study size increases. Small studies scatter more widely at the base of the graph. So, visual examination of the plot should reveal in the absence of bias a triangular or symmetrical, inverted funnel shape. Departure from this shape may be due to bias. Other explanations may include the low quality of small studies; heterogeneity; and chance. Discuss this in the Discussion section of the review. Bias will most likely be in a positive direction.

Table 3.3 (Continued)

Synthesize data

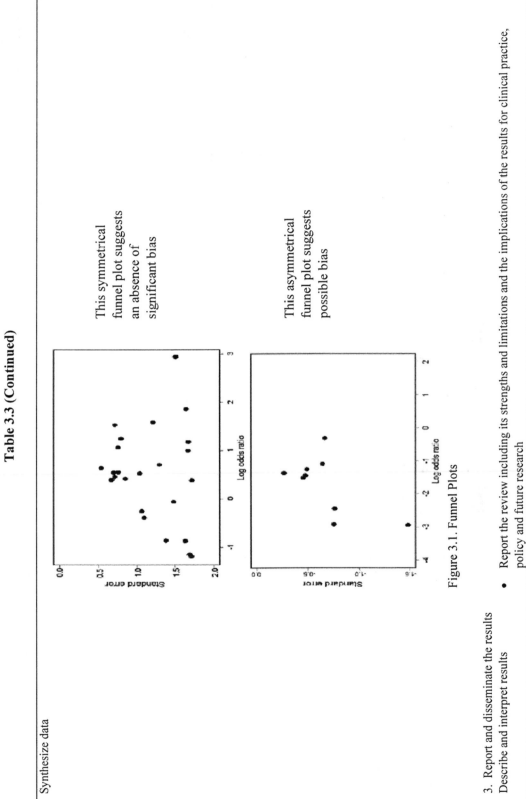

This symmetrical funnel plot suggests an absence of significant bias

This asymmetrical funnel plot suggests possible bias

Figure 3.1. Funnel Plots

3. Report and disseminate the results
Describe and interpret results

• Report the review including its strengths and limitations and the implications of the results for clinical practice, policy and future research

Table 3.4. Assessing the Degree and Impact of Heterogeneity

Steps to take	Description
Look for clinical heterogeneity	Explore the influences of specific clinical differences between the individual studies
Make a visual assessment of statistical heterogeneity	Produce a forest plot (Figure 3.2) to display results from the individual studies on a common scale. Heterogeneity is suggested when the confidence intervals of different studies overlap poorly or not at all; the weight is the influence given to each study for a pooled analysis

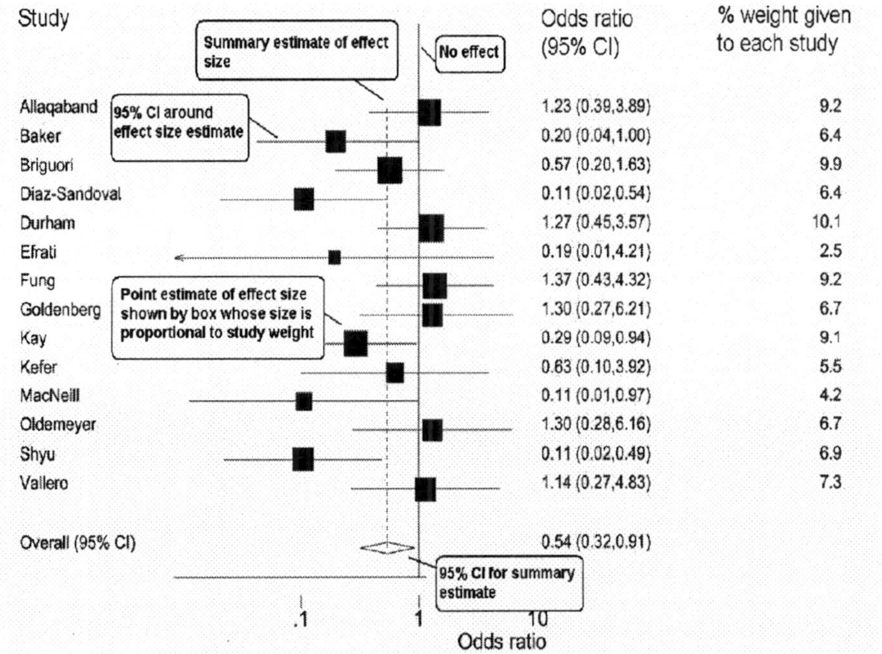

Source: Bagshaw SM, Ghali WA. Acetylcysteine for prevention of contrast-induced nephropathy after intravascular angiography: a systematic review and meta-analysis. *BMC Med 2004*; 2(1): 38.

Figure 3.2. Forest Plot

Table 3.4 (Continued)

The L'Abbé scatter plot (Figure 3.3) can also reveal heterogeneity between outliers. It maps events rates in the intervention group against event rates in the control group. The points will lie around the diagonal (line of equality) if the effects are homogenous

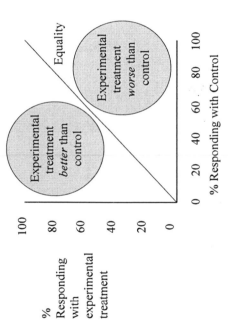

Figure 3.3. L'Abbé plot

Table 3.4 (Continued)

Make a quantitative assessment of statistical heterogeneity	• Identify and measure the degree of heterogeneity
	  Perform a chi-square test for heterogeneity (Cochran's Q test). This test assesses whether the individual study effects differ from the pooled effect more than is expected by chance. Its power to detect heterogeneity is small when the numbers of studies, or the sample sizes, are small. So if $p < 0.10$, conclude that significant heterogeneity is present. If the number of studies is large, the test has high power to reveal a little heterogeneity that may lack clinical importance
	• Address the heterogeneity
	  If we find heterogeneity, consider these options:
	  1. Check the data
	  2. Change the effect measure
	  3. Explore potential reasons for the heterogeneity:
	    a. Calculate summary measures for each subgroup defined at the outset (subgroup analysis)
	    b. Calculate summary measures omitting one study at a time (influence analysis)
	    c. Assess the ability of study characteristics to account for the effect estimate from individual studies (meta-regression); ideally, analyze individuals' data rather than summary data
	  4. Perform a meta-analysis (Tables 3.5-3.7)
	    a. Perform a random effects meta-analysis to incorporate *unexplained* heterogeneity across the studies
	    b. Ignore the heterogeneity through a fixed effects meta-analysis to test the (null) hypothesis of no effect in every study
	  5. Do not perform a meta-analysis; produce a narrative synthesis

Statistical assessment of impact of heterogeneity	Perform Higgins I^2 test to estimate the percentage of the inconsistency in effect estimates due to heterogeneity rather than sampling error

Table 3.5. Approaches to Evidence Synthesis

Type of review with which each approach is typically associated	General approach to synthesis	Type of synthesis	Description	Rationale	Purpose	Method	Advantages	Disadvantages
Narrative	Narrative review	Narrative summary	Narrative description and ordering of evidence	Variation and gaps in the evidence (e.g. for successful programmes)	Identify patterns and directions in the evidence	Infers the package of attributes that produce positive outcomes	See Table 3.2	
Systematic	Descriptive	Qualitative	Tabulation of characteristics and results of included studies, wherefrom differences between these studies can be qualitatively assessed	Variation in study characteristics, quality and results	Plan quantitative syntheses and whether participants, interventions and outcomes allow review findings to be generalized	Systematic qualitative assessment of the evidence (See Tables 3.3 and 3.4)	See Tables 3.3 and 3.4	
		Narrative	Descriptive and interpretative synthesis of the main, common or recurrent findings across multiple primary studies	Disparate evidence. Need to help decision makers configure interventions to be like successful ones	Generate new, knowledge and insights, typically on 'exemplary cases'	Systematic analytical approach involving words and text. Thematic analysis is typical. Also conceptual mapping and summary tables	Flexible, yet more systematic, and transparent than the narrative review. Can combine different types of evidence (research and non-research)	Limited use thus far, so few examples exist

Table 3.5 (Continued)

Type of review	General approach to synthesis	Type of synthesis	Description	Rationale	Purpose	Method	Advantages	Disadvantages
	Qualitative	Cross-case analysis (also called comparative case method or comparative analysis) [10]. Includes meta-ethnography [11 12]	Interpretative synthesis (reconceptualization) of written qualitative findings from whole comparable cases across studies	Opportunity to develop new, conceptually innovative knowledge cumulatively by comparing cases	Inductively produce new insights on a particular issue or concept from existing studies. Meta-ethnography aims to develop a higher order theory	Qualitatively re-analyses and systematically compares purposively selected qualitative (and potentially quantitative) case findings from different studies	Yields a new interpretation, which can account for, and potentially synthesize, divergent quantitative and qualitative results	Yields only one of different interpretations. Need for comparable cases. Low potential for full qualitative-quantitative synthesis. Complex approach requiring experience in use
	Quantitative	Methods such as the case survey and manifest content analysis	Conversion and synthesis of qualitative data, aggregated and derived from different studies, for statistical analysis	Generate aggregative and 'objective' knowledge and understanding of a particular issue	Move beyond the particular case and, in content analysis, test hypotheses	Systematically codes and converts text from different studies into data for statistical analysis	Systematic and straightforward approach to qualitative-quantitative synthesis of text across studies	Qualitatively reductionist. Content analysis emphasizes what is countable rather than important
		Formal statistical techniques such as meta-analysis (Table 3.6)	Comparison and combination of the statistical results of included studies	Heterogeneity, bias and limitations of individual studies (see 3.6)	Assess size and consistency of effect sizes across studies, and perform a meta-analysis if appropriate	Statistical methods for assessing variation in study findings and pooling results (See 3.4 and 3.6)	See Tables 3.3 to 3.7	

Table 3.5 (Continued)

Type of review	General approach to synthesis	Type of synthesis	Description	Rationale	Purpose	Method	Advantages	Disadvantages
Realist	Realist [3 13]	Explanatory model of research synthesis for complex social interventions	Need to refine theory and so offer relevant and timely evidence for decision support	Increase understanding of how complex interventions work or not, under what conditions, and with what effect	Generate programme theories	Understand how the programme mechanism and context yield an outcome pattern	New approach, yet it requires experienced use. Yields tentative findings. Potential for relativism	

Table 3.6. Conducting a Meta-Analysis

Aim	Analyze statistically the summary results from all relevant, independent studies. If possible, produce a single statistical estimate of the effect of the intervention or exposure by pooling the individual effects reported in separate (experimental or observational; see Figure 2.1 and Table 2.2) combinable studies

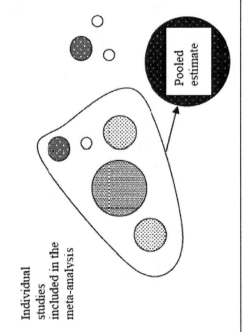

Individual studies included in the meta-analysis

Pooled estimate

Table 3.6 (Continued)

Purpose	• Exclude bias (systematic error) • Increase the statistical power to detect a real effect, as statistically significant • Increase the precision of estimates of the effect • Address new questions not posed by individual studies • Assess the amount of variability between studies • Be transparent in decisions taken • Moderate conflicting results from different studies
Rationale	• Many studies of effect result in uncertainty, owing for example to their small size, and conflict in their estimate of net effect: some show benefit, others harm
Requirements	• High quality systematic review • Effect estimates reported in more than one study • No study characteristics (e.g. biases) and differences between studies that are likely to make comparisons meaningless and distort a pooled result significantly • Common outcome measurement • Lack of significant heterogeneity between studies
Process	1. Produce a systematic review, as in Table 3.3 2. Decide on comparisons to make for the purpose of the meta-analysis 3. Decide whether to produce a summary (pooled) estimate of the effects estimated in these studies. If necessary and possible, address evidence of significant heterogeneity between studies (Table 3.4) 4. Produce a pooled estimate, if appropriate (Table 3.7). Interpret the findings: discuss what they mean and how much confidence can be placed in this meaning
Advantages	Can systematically produce a single, 'objective,' precise and relatively unbiased estimate of effect on a common scale, using all the research evidence available
Disadvantages	The usefulness of meta-analysis depends on the quality of the studies included and the validity of unproven assumptions (e.g. that it is reasonable to generalize beyond individual studies). Application of the methodology must also be correct [14 15] so as not to lose key differences between the studies.

Table 3.7. Producing Pooled Estimates of Effect

Type of meta-analysis	If we find no real evidence of heterogeneity, or we can address the heterogeneity in a manner that makes meta-analysis suitable, we can consider which type of meta-analysis to use. We can pool the effect estimates in one step (standard meta-analysis) or repeat performance of the meta-analysis (cumulative meta-analysis) by adding one study at a time, as it becomes available to include, in order to reveal new trends early and continue to give updated estimates of effect
Outcomes	How we express effect sizes will depend on the type of outcome data • Continuous outcomes: express effect sizes as mean differences between the study groups (when studies report the outcome on the same scale) or as standardized mean differences (when studies use different scales) • Dichotomous outcomes: effects are typically expressed as odds ratios or relative risks
Method of pooling effects	Pool effect estimates using fixed and/or random effects models, and report one
Assumption	*Fixed effects models* Each study is a random sample of a single population and estimates one true (fixed) effect	*Random effects models* Allow for random variation between-studies (as well as within studies) in assessing the effect of the intervention
Weights. All methods use weighted averages of the treatment effects estimated in individual studies	Largely driven by sample size: a larger study is given more weight Summary results of both models are similar	Smaller and more uniform
Between study variation:		
• A little	Random effect models produce a larger confidence interval around pooled estimates (i.e. more conservative) than do the fixed effect models	
• A lot	Inverse variance method: unsuited to low event rates or small studies	
Common methods	• Mantel-Haenszel method: suited to sparse data for dichotomous outcomes • Peto method: can only pool odds ratios; suited to small treatment effects, low event rates and balanced studies • Bayesian meta-analysis includes qualitative evidence	• DerSimonian and Laird • Bayesian

Meta-Ethnography

We turn now to qualitative synthesis. Table 3.5 introduced the approach of cross-case analysis. Table 3.8 elaborates on one form of this type of analysis: meta-ethnography. The table indicates how to use meta-ethnography qualitatively to synthesize data and construct interpretations across studies. Seven sequential steps are described. In practice, however, these steps are unlikely to be linear. The steps of 'translation' and synthesis, in particular, are iterative.

Table 3.8. Undertaking Meta-Ethnography

Step [7 16 17]	Description
Get started	Identify a research question to address in a synthesis of qualitative (and potentially quantitative) research
Find and select relevant studies	Search for, and purposively select, studies relevant to 'answering' the research question
Read the studies	Peruse the studies to identify key concepts and study details that can aid understanding of the concepts
Determine how the studies are related	Consider relationships between concepts emerging from the different studies; produce a grid to juxtapose concepts from each study against details of the design of each study
Translate the studies into each other	Interpret the interpretations of the studies reporting similar methods and findings (reciprocal translation) or appearing to contradict each other (refutational translation)
Synthesize the translations	Compare these translations to produce inductively a new, general higher-order interpretation grounded in the findings of the individual studies (line of argument synthesis)
Express the synthesis	Communicate the synthesis in a form relevant to the target audience

QUALITY ASSESSMENT

This section refers briefly to methods for the critical appraisal of the quality of systematic reviews and meta-analyses of studies with different designs. The next chapter includes some criteria for evaluating the quality of qualitative research, including meta-ethnography (Table 4.8).

Systematic reviews of randomized controlled trials:
The QUORUM [18] 18-item checklist (Table 3.9) is the 'gold standard' for defining the quality of reporting of systematic reviews and meta-analyses of randomized controlled trials. It offers a comprehensive guideline as well as a tool for reviewing existing reports of systematic reviews. It also describes the materials to be included in each report of a meta-analysis.

Systematic reviews of observational studies:
The Meta-analysis Of Observational Studies in Epidemiology (MOOSE) [19] checklist summarizes 35 recommendations for reporting meta-analyses of observational studies.

Table 3.9. QUORUM (Quality of Reporting of Meta-analyses) checklist for randomized trials

Heading	Subheading	Descriptor
Title		Identify the report as a meta-analysis (or systematic review of randomized trials)
Abstract		Use a structured format
		Describe:
	Objectives	• The clinical question explicitly
	Data sources	• The databases (i.e. list) and other information sources
	Review methods	• The selection criteria (i.e. population, intervention, outcome, and study design); methods for validity assessment, data abstraction, and study characteristics, and quantitative data synthesis in sufficient detail to permit replication
	Results	• Characteristics of the randomized trials included and excluded; qualitative and quantitative findings (i.e. point estimates and confidence intervals); and sub-group analyses
	Conclusion	• The main results
		Describe:
Introduction		• The explicit clinical problem, biological rationale for the intervention and rationale for the review
Methods	Searching	• The information sources in detail (e.g. databases, registers, personal files, expert informants, agencies, hand-searching), and any restrictions (years considered, publication status, language of publication)
	Selection	• The inclusion and exclusion criteria (defining population, intervention, principal outcomes, and study design)
	Validity assessment	• The criteria and process used (e.g. masked conditions, quality assessment, and their findings)
	Data abstraction	• The process or processes used (e.g. completed independently, in duplicate)
	Study characteristics	• The type of study design, participants' characteristics, details of intervention, outcome definitions, and how clinical heterogeneity was assessed
	Quantitative data synthesis	• The principal measures of effect (e.g. relative risk), method of combining results (statistical testing and confidence intervals), handling of missing data; how statistical heterogeneity was assessed; a rationale for any a priori sensitivity and sub-group analyses; and any assessment of publication bias
Results	Trial flow	Provide a meta-analysis profile summarizing trial flow
	Study characteristics	Present descriptive data for each trial (e.g. age, sample size, intervention, dose, duration, follow-up period)
	Quantitative data synthesis	Report agreement on the selection and validity assessment; present simple summary results (for each treatment group in each trial, for each primary outcome); data needed to calculate effect sizes and confidence intervals in intention-to-treat analyses (e.g. 2 * 2 tables of counts, means and standard deviations, proportions)
Discussion		Summarize key findings; discuss clinical inferences based on internal and external validity; interpret the results in the light of the totality of available evidence; describe potential biases in the review process (e.g. publication bias); and suggest a future research agenda

MAKING PRACTICAL USE OF REVIEWS AND EVIDENCE SYNTHESES

Unease has grown over the relevance of systematic reviews and meta-analyses to decision-making in real-world settings – e.g. policy development, management, and patient settings. This concern has led to new realist models (Tables 3.2 and 3.5), which go beyond questions of 'what works?' to attempts to elucidate 'why' and 'how' in specific settings. Other responses have included guidance for applying in clinical practice the results of systematic reviews and meta-analyses (Table 3.10).

**Table 3.10. Applying Results of Systematic
Reviews and Meta-Analyses in Clinical practice**

Are the results of the systematic review generalizable to my patients?	• Expect some variation between individual patients and the patients described in systematic reviews. However, differences in effect tend to be of degree rather than direction. They may also be unimportant (e.g. independent of differences in pathogenesis) or remediable (e.g. by adjusting drug dosages to patient responsiveness). Observational studies are important in assessing the applicability of group findings
Is the intervention feasible to use in practice?	• Assess whether the intervention reviewed is locally accessible

What is the clinical benefit: risk ratio for my patients?	• Derive clinical estimates of the average effect of the intervention on patients at the average risk in the studies reviewed; i.e. calculate the Number Needed to Treat (NNT) to prevent one clinical event, and its confidence interval (and/or the Number Needed to Harm, NNH)
	 • Consider using the aggregate ratio, 'the Likelihood of Being Helped or Harmed' [20]
	 • Extrapolate estimates to the individual patient. Options include:
	   1. Extrapolating from the most relevant subgroups defined at the outset
	   2. Using multivariate risk prediction equations
	   3. Dividing the NNT (and NNH) by:
	     a. a factor (f) that relates the risk in the individual patient, according to clinical judgment, to that of the average patient in the review; and
	     b. Ratings by individual patients of their valuations (utilities) of the help and harm resulting from the treatment

How can I incorporate patient values and preferences?	• Use decision aids to help elicit informed preferences, and make shared decisions that reflect the patient perspective

REFERENCES

[1]   Sheldon T. Making evidence synthesis more useful. *J. Health Serv. Res. Policy* 2005;10(Suppl 1):S1:1-S1:5.

[2]   Whittemore R, Knafl K. The integrative review: updated methodology. *J. Adv. Nurs.* 2005;52:546-53.

[3]   Pawson R, Greenhalgh T, Harvey G, Walshe K. Realist review - a new method of systematic review designed for complex policy interventions. *J. Health Serv. Res. Policy* 2005;10(Suppl 1):S1:21-S1:34.

[4]   Egger M, Davey Smith G, Altman D, editors. *Systematic Reviews in Health Care*. London: BMJ Books, 2003.

[5]   Higgins J, Green S (eds). *Cochrane Handbook for Systematic Reviews of Interventions 4.2.5* [updated May 2005], 2005.

[6]   Hopewell S, McDonald S, Clarke M, Egger M. Grey literature in meta-analyses of randomized trials of health care interventions. *The Cochrane Database of Systematic Reviews* 2005(3).

[7]   Noblitt G, Hare R. *Meta-ethnography: Synthesising Qualitative Studies*. Newbury Park: Sage, 1988.

[8]   Lomas J, Culyer T, McCutcheon C, McAuley L, Law S, for the Canadian Health Services Research Foundation. *Final Report. Conceptualizing and Combining Evidence for Health System Guidance*. Ottawa: Canadian Health Services Research Foundation, 2005.

[9]   Mays N, Pope C, Popay J. Systematically reviewing qualitative and quantitative evidence to inform management and policy-making in the health field. *J. Health Serv. Res. Policy* 2005;10(Suppl 1):S1:6-S1:20.

[10]   Ragin C. *The Comparative Method: Moving Beyond Qualitative and Quantitative Strategies*. Berkeley: University of California Press, 1987.

[11]   Schwandt T. *Dictionary of Qualitative Inquiry*. 2nd Edition. Thousand Oaks: Sage Publications, 2001.

[12]   Campbell R, Britten N, Pound P, Donovan J, Morgan M, Pill R, et al. Using meta-ethnography to synthesise qualitative research. . In: Popay P (ed). *Moving beyond effectiveness in evidence synthesis. Methodological issues in the synthesis of diverse sources of evidence*. London: National Institute for Health and Clinical Excellence, 2006:75-82.

[13]   Pawson R. Evidence-based policy: The promise of 'realist synthesis'. *Evaluation* 2002;8:340-58.

[14]   Eysenck H. Problems with meta-analysis. In: Chalmers I, Altman D (eds). *Systematic Reviews*. London: *BMJ* Publishing Group, 1995:64-74.

[15]   Bailar J. The promise and problems of meta-analysis. *N. Eng. J. Med.* 1997;337:559-60.

[16]   Britten N, Campbell R, Pope C, Donovan J, Morgan M, Pill R. Using meta ethnography to synthesise qualitative research: a worked example. *J. Health Serv. Res. Policy* 2002;7:209-15.

[17]   Doyle L. Synthesis through meta-ethnography: paradoxes, enhancements, and possibilities. *Qual. Res.* 2003;3(3):321-44.

[18]   Moher D, Cook D, Eastwood S, Olkin I, Rennie D, Stroup D. Improving the quality of reports of meta-analyses of randomised controlled trials: the QUOROM statement. Quality of Reporting of Meta-analyses. *Lancet* 1999;354:1896-1900.

[19]   Stroup D, Berlin J, Morton S, Olkin I, Williamson G, Rennie D, et al. Meta-analysis of observational studies in epidemiology: a proposal for reporting. Meta-analysis Of Observational Studies in Epidemiology (MOOSE) group. *JAMA* 2000;283:2008-12.

[20]   Straus SE. Individualizing treatment decisions. The likelihood of being helped or harmed. *Eval Health Professions* 2002;25:210-24.

Chapter 4

QUALITATIVE RESEARCH

OBJECTIVES

By the time you have completed this chapter, you should be able to:

1. Describe characteristics of, and ethical issues in, qualitative research
2. Report different sampling strategies for qualitative research
3. Summarize different approaches to gathering, processing, analyzing and reporting qualitative data
4. Know how to enhance and evaluate the quality of qualitative research

PREVIEW

Chapter 1 introduced qualitative research, comparing its general nature and purposes to those of quantitative research. This chapter begins by elaborating on defining characteristics of qualitative research and its particular ethical risks and strategies. The chapter then comments briefly on qualitative study plans before focusing on the methodological skills that are needed to undertake qualitative research. In this context, sampling options will be described before consideration is given to how to collect, process, analyze and present or report qualitative data. For the sake of clarity the chapter discusses these stages in sequence but it should be emphasized that in practice the different stages are frequently concurrent and iterative. Strategies to enhance and evaluate the different types of qualitative health research are noted last.

CHARACTERISTICS

Qualitative research methodology is appropriate if the principal purpose of the research is to describe and understand the meaning of human and social action, and its significance in context-specific, natural settings. Qualitative research can help to advance the never-ending journey toward understanding the world, through its characteristic focus on 'bricolage' (Table 4.1)

Table 4.1. Qualitative Research Characteristics

- Bricolage [1], a collage-like 'gluing' together of constructed representations through the creative use of interdisciplinary and multi-method practices
- Respect for the uniqueness and integrity of the information-rich experiences of the participants and researcher(s)
- Interpretation through intuition, sense-making, reflexivity (critical self-reflection), and ownership of one's own perspective and voice
- Context-sensitivity to the situated meaning of what is being studied
- Observables including an empirical orientation to study cases (e.g. individuals, groups programs or events) from which generalizations to concepts or models can be made
- Lebenswelt, meaning the natural world that people experience and live in
- Action-orientation toward empathetic, inter-subjective understanding of peoples' intentions and goal-oriented, purposive behavior
- Gestalt, meaning a holistic perspective
- Emergent research designs that evolve during the study in response to the researcher's developing understanding of, or change in, the study setting

ETHICAL ISSUES

Ethical issues characterize all health research. However, with its probing search for in-depth understanding, qualitative research faces particular ethical risks of harming participants [2]. For some practitioners – influenced, for example, by critical theory – qualitative research also imposes a moral responsibility to use the research to help improve participants' lives and transform society. To avoid harm and possibly help participants, Table 4.2 therefore summarizes the most important ethical risks in qualitative research and suggests how best to manage them with Ethics approval.

STUDY PLANS

There are no prescribed designs for qualitative research [3]. However, all qualitative research requires careful planning and some combination of theory and empirical evidence in order to fashion an argument that can address the study question or study problem. According to Mason [4], plans for qualitative research respond to three broad questions: (1) What is the planned research about? (2) How will it link the study question with the methods used and evidence collected? (3) How will the research accommodate pertinent ethical and political concerns? More fundamentally, Chapter 1 considered metatheories that may underpin the choice of study question and the methodology used to answer it; and Table 1.5 described the central question and principal methods of key methodologies relevant to conducting qualitative research. These methodologies vary greatly but include grounded theory, phenomenology and ethnography. Other common qualitative methodologies include a general inductive approach. It uses the study aims to identify topics to investigate before identifying core meanings or summary themes from close readings and interpretations of the raw data. Subsequent sections of this chapter consider issues relevant to the general and specific application of planned qualitative research.

Table 4.2. Ethics in Qualitative Research: Risk and Strategies

Risk	Strategy to manage risk, requiring Ethics approval
Anxiety or distress in participants	• Provide the information and support that participants can reasonably expect before, during and after the data collection
	• Consider seeking verbal consent where participants in sensitive research may feel highly vulnerable and fear being identified. The study should involve no more than minimal risk to them
	• Ask to waive the requirement to seek consent when it is impossible to seek consent from all participants (e.g. in some ethnographic research) or when seeking consent for very low-risk research would act against the need for naturalistic inquiry
Exploitation	• Ensure that the research is scientifically sound, clear, relevant, and respectful of the participants
	• Usually seek free and informed written consent, which participants can withhold or withdraw at any time without risk to their health care
	• Minimize the costs to participants as far as possible
	• Separate the roles of researcher and clinician
Misinterpretation	• Consider involving two or more researchers in the data analysis
	• Be reflexive and acknowledge how personal and professional attributes may influence the research
Misrepresentation	• Solicit feedback from participants about your findings (informant checking; also called member checking and member or respondent validation). This can generate data and insight about, for example, the defensibility of the findings
Not protecting participants' confidentiality and anonymity	• Discuss limits to confidentiality; e.g. the Law may require disclosure. Confidentiality cannot be guaranteed in focus groups
	• Store tapes and transcripts securely
	• Keep identifying details separate from the data and all reports

SAMPLING STRATEGIES

Qualitative research typically focuses on small samples in which information-rich participants are selected purposively to represent and produce in-depth understanding of the particular issue or phenomenon of interest (e.g. experience of having an illness). Purposive sampling (also called purposeful, selective or judgment sampling) selects the participants who are most relevant to answering the research question. This sampling is deliberately 'biased' in order to identify efficiently only the participants who have the most experience and are able to communicate it. Purposive sampling differs from the strategy of random sampling as used in quantitative research to select samples representative of the population from which the sample was drawn. Random samples are inefficient for understanding a phenomenon through qualitative research. They include participants other than just those who can best represent the phenomenon of interest. Random samples tend, therefore, to be overlarge (which does not suit the bulky nature of qualitative data), and to produce too much data on some things and too little data on others [5].

Table 4.3 summarizes a menu of useful strategies for purposive sampling [6]. Qualitative researchers choose a strategy relevant to their research question and, consistent with this strategy, set criteria for selecting individual participants (e.g., those who have survived a stroke; can understand spoken English; can speak English) and the sample group (e.g., varies by age and gender). We are able to continue to review our criteria while collecting qualitative data.

Table 4.3. Purposive Sampling Strategies

Strategies	Method
Theoretical sampling	Select the sample in an ongoing manner on the basis of the theory that emerges from concurrent collection and analysis of data. (Some people distinguish theoretical sampling from purposive sampling, arguing that the latter is decided before the onset of data collection whereas the former is not) [7]
Maximum variation (heterogeneity) sampling	Select a diverse range of participants who can represent common themes that cut across the variation in the sample. Describing the participants in detail can document uniqueness
Stratified purposeful sampling	Select different sub-samples of interest (each of which is reasonably homogenous) in order to represent major variation rather than a common perspective
Homogeneous sampling	Select similar participants to increase the focus of the study
Critical participant sampling	Select participants who can signify ideally what is possible or not possible and therefore make logical generalizations possible
Typical participant sampling	Select 'typical' or average participants whose experiences are illustrative
Intensity sampling	Select participants who represent some phenomenon of interest intensely but not extremely; for example, good rather than exceptional nurses
Extreme participant sampling	Identify and select participants at some extreme whose experience is edifying
Unique participant sampling	Identify and select participants with rare attributes of interest

DATA COLLECTION

Data are not necessarily 'out there' to be located and assembled without contamination in order to reveal true meanings. Data may instead be constructed through the researcher supporting participants to bring understanding and meaning into focus. What constitutes 'data' depends therefore on the purpose of the research and on the questions posed within theoretical schemes that justify particular methodological approaches [3]. This section describes and evaluates key approaches that can be taken to collect, or gather, data to meet particular purposes in qualitative research. Table 4.4 focuses mainly on the strategies of observation; interviewing; note-taking; and document gathering. Some of the strategies discussed also characterize other types of research but they are considered in the Table in the context of their use in qualitative health research. At the risk of over-simplification, Table 4.5 summarizes descriptive characteristics that further distinguish between the use of personal interviews and one type of group interview – focus groups – as qualitative research methods for data gathering.

Table 4.4. Strategies for Collecting Qualitative Data

Type	Subtype	Purpose	Method	Strengths	Weaknesses
Observation	Self-observations and reflexivity	Help us become critically self-aware of, and own, how our perspective and voice vis-à-vis the perspectives of others shapes our research	Require us to reflect critically on our own assumptions and agendas in analyzing other people's accounts of their lives	Situate the 'I' in qualitative research and enable high quality research sensitive to how the researcher behaves	Can be difficult to learn and practice. Risk producing narcissism, self-righteousness and nihilism
	Simple observations	Describe and discover natural occurrences of events that participants may be unaware of or unwilling to discuss	View participants in their 'natural setting.' The observer role may be known by all, some or none of the participants.	Can use unobtrusive measures to reveal directly what really happens. Observation provides a check on other sources of data	Focus on external behavior. Risk participants behaving differently if they know they are being observed. Covert observation may be unethical
	Participant observations	As above, but provide an insider (emic) perspective which, for example allows empathy to help uncover the meaning of situations	Involve us collaboratively as 'members' of the study group who can observe this group from the inside in its natural context	Can offer first-hand insights on naturally occurring (including deviant) and unexpected behavior. Can combine different data collection methods at the same time	Can be time consuming and incomplete. Can require negotiation of the degree of participation that is possible and acceptable
Note-taking (in your diary or note book); also as a means of data recording	Descriptive field notes	Aid our own and others' understanding of the field setting, what is happening there and what it means	Keep an ongoing record, which concretely describes field observations and experiences. Best to complete at the site	Aid the recall of, and focus on, salient events. Provides useful background and contextual information.	May distract the participant and researcher, during interviews. Risk inaccuracies if special skills are absent
	Personal (reflective) notes	Clarify our own thoughts and experiences. Provide a contextual framework for interpreting our descriptive field notes	Maintain a record of personal reflections on our feelings, our insights and what we are learning during the fieldwork	Aid the process of starting to interpret the personal meaning, causes and significance of events	Require researchers to avoid imposing preconceptions and premature judgments during fieldwork

Table 4.4 (Continued)

Type	Subtype	Purpose	Method	Strengths	Weaknesses
	Method notes	Record thoughts about the usefulness of certain methods, their effects, and how to achieve improvements	Describe the methods used; the reasons; and why any changes were made during field work	Strengthen evidence of using rigorous (trustworthy) methods during fieldwork to yield high quality data	As above
	Theory notes	Develop emergent analytic propositions and hypotheses as part of theory building	Document developing hypotheses, ideas and connections with the study's theoretical framework	Produce beginning analyses of our observations and experiences, which can be further developed	As above
Self-complete questionnaires	Self-complete structured survey questionnaires (including postal, mail and on-line questionnaires) with open questions	Obtain responses to a the same broad set of completely specified questions of predetermined interest to the researcher	Produce and administer a questionnaire for participants' independent self-completion and return	Are relatively unobtrusive and low cost. Make it relatively easy to collect and analyze a broad range of anonymized data, free of interviewer bias and standardized to aid participant comparability	Are ill-suited to participants with low literacy and to obtaining deep data on complex issues. Cannot probe and offer little flexibility. Often yield low response rates. Often leave researchers uncertain who has returned questionnaires by mail, fax or the internet
Documents (written texts)	Primary, secondary and tertiary documents	Reveal or help to verify information that varies according to the vantage of the author	Include primary documents, produced by participants or witnesses; secondary documents, written by others after an event; and tertiary documents (e.g. internet search engines) to aid the location of references	Provide a potentially low-cost, rich and stable source of information about past and present events that may not be directly observable	Can make it necessary to authenticate primary and tertiary documents. Primary documents can be difficult to read and understand in context. Secondary and tertiary documents may be incomplete and inaccurate

Table 4.4 (Continued)

Type	Subtype	Purpose	Method	Strengths	Weaknesses
	Public and private documents	Reveal information using sources that may vary according to their degree of accessibility	Include public and private documents that may be closed, restricted, open-archival or open-published	As above.	As above. Access to private documents may be limited. The release of damaging, private details can produce a backlash
	Solicited and unsolicited documents	Reveal insights from texts produced for research purposes or personal use	Include, when solicited, documents produced with the research in mind. Unsolicited documents are intended for personal use but address an audience	Can use solicited documents that tend to be the most directly relevant to the research for which they were produced.	As above. Personal documents can be especially difficult to interpret. Solicited documents may lack authenticity
Interviews Degree of formality and structure [8]	Informal conversational interviews (also called depth, unstructured or ethnographic interviews)	Explore directions taken by participants and the data	Explore one or two issues conversationally and in depth with no other predetermined structure	Aid participant candor. Flexible and responsive to situational and individual differences	Can be time consuming, not dependable, require highly skilled interviewers, and be difficult to analyze
	Semi-structured interviews	Elucidate and illuminate a subject area predetermined by the researcher	Use an interview guide which outlines general topics and issues to probe and explore. Decide on the wording and sequence of questions during the interviews	Balance the need for a flexible, but also systematic, approach	Can omit relevant topics. Interviewer flexibility can reduce the comparability of participant responses

Table 4.4 (Continued)

Type	Subtype	Purpose	Method	Strengths	Weaknesses
	Structured interviews with open questions	Obtain responses in depth to the same set of completely specified questions of predetermined interest to the researcher	Use an interview schedule to ask the same questions (including open questions), in the same order, predetermined by the researcher	Permit the pre-screening of questions. Maximize the comparability of responses. Minimize interviewer effects. Facilitate analysis	Lack flexibility in making the interview relevant to participants in their situation
Number interviewed at the same time	Personal (one-to-one) interviews	Collect personal data	Use an interviewer to interview each participant separately	Permit an intense and safe focus on the views of each participant	Are resource intensive
	Group interviews (e.g. focus groups, nominal groups, Delphi groups, observations of naturally occurring groups)	Use group interaction to generate broad data	Use one or two interviewers together to interview a group	Permit participants to consider their viewpoints cognizant of the views of others in social interaction. Can identify major themes	Are cost-effective. Multiple audiences can produce bias. Are unsuited to sensitive discussions and microanalysis. Cannot guarantee confidentiality
Mode of administration	Face to face interviews	Collect depth data of high response quality from participants in person	Collect interview data, using potentially diverse data collecting strategies, in one place at one time	Typically achieve high participation rates. Suited to open questions, with physical prompts and probes. Can detect non-verbal cues. Conducive to thoughtful responses	Are expensive, slow and time-consuming. The presence of the interviewer may be biasing
	Telephone interviews	Gather information cost-effectively from a geographically dispersed sample	Conduct interviews on the telephone	Are low cost, quick and able to reach geographically dispersed participants. Generally achieve good response rates. Computer assisted personal interviews can aid conduct and analysis	May involve samples that are unrepresentative. No observation. Can limit the types of questions posed. Participants can hang up

Table 4.4 (Continued)

Type	Subtype	Purpose	Method	Strengths	Weaknesses
	Computer-mediated interviews: includes online synchronous interviews, online asynchronous interviews and virtual focus groups	Collect high quality qualitative data quickly and at low cost from participants who may otherwise be difficult to access	Use the internet to conduct and directly record interviews	Are low cost, fast and suited to asking sensitive questions of large numbers of people, including hard-to-reach participants, over large geographical distances. Can use graphics and visual aids. Eliminate transcription costs	Need shared access to, and knowledge of, an internet, browser and software. Responses can be cryptic and lack depth. May involve no access to aural and other bodily cues to aid rapport and interpretation [9]. Coverage error is a threat, especially in surveys [10]
What happens during interviews	Neutral interviews	Gain direct and disinterested access to participants' experiences	Collect interview data as a verbal exchange that aims to ask the right questions to elicit authentic responses	Use interviewer detachment to minimize bias, and produce clean, comprehensive data that speak for themselves, facilitating their analysis	Can become a pastiche produced by fiat, isolated from their social context, and claiming an illusory neutrality
	Active interviews [11 12]	Contextualize the negotiated meanings of questions and responses	Recognize that interviews, are non-neutral social encounters (in which interviewers actively participate) and collect data as negotiated text that constructs joint meanings	Can be used morally, reflexively and politically to advance the interests of participants and interviewers	May fail when reciprocity of perspective does not exist. Findings can be used against the study group
Interviewing approach: linkage between philosophy and method	Phenomenological interviews [13]	Uncover through direct description the structure and meaning of participants' lived experience of some phenomenon (as it appears in their consciousness)	Ask interviewers to suspend and set aside (bracket) their own preunderstandings. Participants are asked to describe their own concrete experiences of the study phenomenon	Take a cognitive and 'scientific' approach to seeing phenomena as they are through words	Can be challenging to conduct. Bracketing is difficult, if not impossible. Descriptions may not be pre-reflective or may deny participants' interpretations

Table 4.4 (Continued)

Type	Subtype	Purpose	Method	Strengths	Weaknesses
	Hermeneutic phenomenological interviews	Seek to understand what it means to *be* human situated in the world	Expect interviewers and participants to mobilize their preunderstandings and lived experiences as they negotiate the interpretative process	Let participants reflect on the meaning of their experience. Produce close, open involvement of the interviewer, who co-creates the interview	See no false judgments, which relativizes meaning. Pose unavoidable risks to the neutrality of the research. Depends on interviewer self-reflexivity for their credibility.
	Hermeneutic interviews [14]	Co-create meaning and understanding through interpretation of what takes place through language	Permit participants to talk about what they want: Disallow the interviewer to have predetermined questions or presumptions about what matters: meaning arises in language through the dialectic of question and answer	Allow understanding to proceed through, rather than on the basis of, the interviewer's pre-understandings. This keeps opens the possibility of different understandings	Are difficult to conduct. Devalue the contribution of the researcher in the dialogue. May find that researchers cannot suspend their pre-understandings, disabling attempts to be open to new understandings
	Grounded theory interviews [13]	Generate theory	May be informal and formal. The latter begin as relatively unstructured, becoming progressively focused and structured as theory develops	Enable interviews to become progressively focused as theory emerges during the course of the research	Can see interviews become less open as they become shaped by emerging theory
	Narrative interviews [15]	Use recounted stories of individual experience vividly to reconstruct social events and enhance understanding of their situated meanings	Are unstructured or semi-structured interviews that invite participants to tell their own stories, uninterrupted, except to preserve the story flow	Give voice in context to different perspectives, including those that may be otherwise excluded, and their multiple layers	Are at risk of stories' inherent subjectivity, inconsistency and emotionality

Table 4.4 (Continued)

Type	Subtype	Purpose	Method	Strengths	Weaknesses
	Ethnographic interviews [16 17], including naturalistic story gathering [15]	Discover meanings within cultural groups	Are informal interviews with an explicit purpose. Give explanations and pose three sequential types of questions: descriptive, structural and contrast	Contribute inductively to an in-depth naturalistic understanding of different cultures. Scope to produce 'thick description' – multilayered interpretations of social action in context	Are time-consuming, particularistic and costly. Risk over-identification with informants
	Gendered interviews [12]	Minimize gendered differences and elicit an increased range of responses and insights	Involve interviewers and participants of the same gender, each of whom share their power and knowledge and values	Avoid male-female power differences. Acknowledge effects of membership and individuality. Allow the expression of gendered traits	May not recognize that other personal attributes, e.g. ethnicity, also filter knowledge. Some participants may not prefer an interviewer of the same gender as themselves

Table 4.5. Comparison of Focus Groups and Personal Interviews in Qualitative Research

Attribute	Focus groups [18]	Personal interviews
Number of participants	5-10 participants per group	1 participant per interview
Recruitment	High potential for recruitment problems	Generally recruitment problems are less serious than in focus groups
Number of interviews conducted	4-6 usually sufficient, but depends on the research goals, the diversity of the study population, the use of 'segmentation' (groups comprising particular types of participants) and the level of standardization	5+
Composition	Homogeneous and unacquainted	Not applicable
Duration of each interview	1-2 hours	15 minutes to 2 hours
Number of interviewers per interview	1-2 (1 to moderate the interview; the other to note-take, manage information technology, etc)	1

Table 4.5 (Continued)

Attribute	Focus groups [18]			Personal interviews
Topic focus	Narrow, but participants' comments can elicit discussion topics which might not occur in individual interviews			Variable focus
Design alternatives	Degree of structure or control over:			'Unstructured,' semi-structured or structured
	Questions posed:	Group dynamics:	Type of group:	
	High	High	Tightly structured	
	High	Low	Phenomenological	
	Low	High	Exploratory	
	Low	Low	Loosely structured	
Suitability for sensitive topics	Debatable			High
Issue coverage per interview	Low–medium			Medium–high
Breadth of perspective per interview	High			Low
Likely depth of responses per interview	Low			High
Unit of analysis	Group, individual, and individual within the group			Individual
Financial cost	Low			Typically higher than for focus groups

Table 4.6. Recording Tips

Equipment	• Obtain a reliable tape recorder, ideally with a separate microphone, batteries and spares, and an extension cord. Set the fastest tape speed possible
	• Become comfortable with your equipment
	• Load a good quality, one hour, labeled tape. Keep participant identifiers physically separate from the labeled and dated tapes
	• Pretest the recorder before you go to the interview
At the start of the interview	• Attach the recorder to an electrical outlet if available.
	• Choose a quiet, comfortable setting, free from background noise and interruptions. Settings with soft furniture, curtains and carpet help to absorb noise
	• Put the recorder on a stable surface close to the participant.
	• Test the recorder before you begin the interview. Record a few words from the participant and yourself, and check they are audible.
	• Run the tape for 10 seconds before the interview begins
During the interview	• State the date and time at the start Continue to speak slowly, clearly and loud enough to be recorded
	• Ensure that one person speaks at a time
	• Monitor the participant's voice and, if necessary, ask the participant to speak up or repeat anything that is unclear
	• Avoid noise (such as rustling papers) near the recorder
	• Check the tape operation intermittently
	• If an interruption occurs, state the time and turn off the machine. Restart by stating the time. Say the time at the end of the interview
	• At the end of the interview, pull out the tabs on the tape to avoid recording over the interview
After the interview	• As soon as possible after the interview, transcribe the tapes verbatim.
	• By transcribing the tapes yourself, you become familiar with, and can immerse yourself, in the data. Some participants (such as graduate students) can transcribe their own interviews, under editorial control [19]. On average, a one hour interview takes approximately 4-6 hours to transcribe. Make copies of transcripts to protect against loss
	• An alternative to transcribing is to use clipped audio (and video) files to keep the voice (and image) of participants intact for as long as possible [20]

Recording

On the same theme of interviewing, it is helpful in general to audiotape qualitative interviews in order to preserve a complete and accurate record of what was said during them. Audiotaping requires participants' permission. However, permission may be a condition for inclusion in the study. This can be discussed with potential participants at the outset, although they and the researcher should also know that participants are free to withdraw from the study at any time. Table 4.6 summarizes equipment needs and, for the purpose of producing usable recordings to analyze, suggests practical steps to take before, during and after each interview.

DATA ANALYSIS

Data analysis may be undertaken to summarize, describe and interpret text; link the findings derived from the raw data to the research objectives; develop a model or theory; and enable social transformation. Table 4.7 summarizes the most important methods of analysis. Selected methods that are used commonly in my own discipline of primary health care are summarized in more detail in the Table than are the other methods identified.

Table 4.7. Methods of Qualitative Data Analysis

Type	Subtype	Description
Linguistic and/or investigative	Domain analysis	• Analyze language in a cultural context, often to produce a taxonomy
	Narrative analysis [21]	• Analyze individual stories (what and how participants talk about their experiences and situations) as a whole, focusing on the context of the storytelling; the story structure, development and function; and patterns, and evaluations by all participants, across the stories
	Discourse analysis	• Analyze how people use the language of communication to say something in social interaction and thereby construct meaning
	Conversation analysis	• Analyze in detail the content (or structure) of recorded talk (as a form of discourse) in order to derive meaning from its use in social interaction
	Semiotics	• Analyze how signs (language and symbols) construct and convey meanings in particular contexts
	Critical (depth) hermeneutics	• Penetrate deeply and skeptically the linguistic fabric of the text to expose the 'truth' (freedom from ideological distortions such as power, cultural norms and the unconscious), emancipate individuals from false consciousness and transform society
	Post-structural hermeneutics	• Center (privilege) the text and deconstruct it by exposing and critiquing its critical assumptions, revealing its contradictions and freeing it from ideological distortions. In so doing, reveal an unstable, existential 'truth' in language and enable transformation
Enumerative	Manifest (basic) content analysis [22]	• Deductively test hypotheses about the content of language (as communication) by tallying the number of times that particular words, phrases or themes are used in the text (typically documents)
Iterative	Template approach	• Use a specific *a priori* template or code book (from past studies or theoretical perspectives) systematically to organize the data collected
	Thematic content analysis	• Systematically examine the content of the data to identify themes inductively or deductively. Lists of categories (typologies) may reflect our own understanding (*etic* analysis) or emphasize concepts and terms that participants apply (*emic* analysis; also called *in vivo* coding)

Table 4.7 (Continued)

Type	Subtype	Description
	General inductive approach [23]	• Produce a summary framework that reflects the research objectives (deductive) and key categories or themes that emerge from the raw data (inductive). This involves: 1. Close reading of the text 2. Creation of categories or themes (common patterned segments). The upper level or more general categories are likely to come from the research objectives. Derive lower level or specific categories from multiple readings of the raw data 3. Continuing revision and refinement of the category system. Within each category, search for subtopics, including contradictory points of view and new insights. Relate the categories to participant attributes. Where appropriate, combine or connect categories into an overall framework that addresses the research aims
	Editing approach [24]	• Edit the data by searching for meaningful segments, systematically reducing and reassembling the data until their interpretation is complete
	Grounded theory[25 26]	• Coding (analysis) involves identifying themes inductively (through editing), though not *ab novo*, before using deduction (analysis based on these data and data not fitting the categories) to generate a theory about the relationships between concepts
	1. Classic grounded theory	1. Substantive coding to produce categories and identify their properties through: (a) Open coding: Open up the text through immersion; through constantly comparing incident to incident, and incident to emerging category; and through writing memos; and (b) Selective coding: Delimit the coding around a core variable 2. Theoretical coding: Integrate the selective codes to allow hypotheses and theory to emerge naturally and exclusively from the data [25]
	2. Strauss and Corbin version	1. Open coding: Fracture and label concepts in the data; develop categories in terms of their properties and dimensions; use specific analytic tools to facilitate 'theoretical sensitivity' (i.e. 'see' relevant empirical data with the aid of theoretical concepts) 2. Axial coding: Define the relationships (of categories to each other and their subcategories) which coordinate the axis of the categories 3. Selective coding: Integrate the categories around a core category (and each other) in order to build and refine a theory

Table 4.7 (Continued)

Type	Subtype	Description
	Cross-case analysis [27] (comparative case method or comparative analysis)	• Develop new explanations (or, in meta-ethnography, a new higher order theory) by systematically comparing whole, information-rich and comparable cases, for example through matrices
	Analytic induction	• Start with an hypothesis applicable to all cases of the phenomenon under study (deduction) and, through cross-case analysis (see above), continue to test and modify this hypothesis using 'negative cases' (instances that do not fit the hypothesis) from the ongoing data collected (induction)
	Immersion/crystallization [28]	• Become totally immersed in, and reflect on, the data during or after its collection, to produce inductively an *intuitive* crystallization of the data
	Romanticist hermeneutics	• Interpret the text in its historical and cultural context to recover and reconstruct the thoughts of the participant and so reveal the single truth of original authorial intent
	Transcendental phenomenology [29]	• Undertake three main steps to uncover through descriptive analysis the single, unified meaning (essence) of the objects of people's lived experience as these objects present themselves in pure consciousness (not in these people's representations): 1. *(Transcendental) Phenomenological reduction*: (a) Be reflexive (critically self-reflective); suspend our judgment (the *époche*); and 'bracket' out our presuppositions and extraneous influences (b) Delete repetitive, overlapping and irrelevant statements in order to leave behind 'horizons' that we can cluster into themes (c) Organize the horizons and themes into a textual description of *what* the experience of the study phenomenon entails 2. *Eidetic reduction*: Imagine different possible versions of the study phenomenon. What remains unchanged are structural descriptions of *how* it was experienced 2. *Intuitive Synthesis*: Intuitively integrate these textual and structural descriptions to reveal the single, essential, invariant meaning – or essence – of experience of the study phenomenon

Table 4.7 (Continued)

Type	Subtype	Description
	Hermeneutic phenomenology	• Expand and grow interpretation of the text, through a fusion of the horizons of the researcher and participants, to reveal a hidden existential meaning in the here and now: 1. Read and reread each transcribed interview 2. Reflexively and dialectically converse between our own biases and those of the text, since, for hermeneutic phenomenologists, bias 'is an inescapable condition of being and knowing' and the challenge is to distinguish between enabling and disabling bias [3]. In this context: 1. Find and extract from each transcript the stories that 'stand out' in relation to the research question 2. Rewrite these stories in our own words. Include significant statements 3. Check with the participants that the rewritten story is still their story 4. Gather their meanings together. Circle from the whole to the parts and back to the whole 5. Summarize for readers what the data say. Include the stories that best 'show' themes across participants 6. Draw together selected stories and interpretations. Bring in phenomenological and other notions from the literature to aid a credible interpretation
Subjective	Autoethnography	• Use personal, lived experience and introspection to give voice to reflexive insights, as primary data, into understanding a culture of which one is part
	Heuristic phenomenology [30]	• Perform five stages: 1. Intense personal experience (shared by participants as co-researchers) of the phenomenon under study (immersion) 2. Quiet contemplation (incubation) 3. Illumination, which involving an awakening of awareness 4. Explication of what has awakened in consciousness in order to understand the meaning of the experience 5. Creative synthesis of essential meanings of the experience, which include the researcher's intuitions and personal knowledge and keep participants in tact as persons

DATA DISPLAY

Qualitative data are most commonly displayed as extended text (e.g. field notes, transcripts, memos and reports). This text describes the data, and aids the data interpretation and the communication of key findings in a written report. (Quotes are typically included to support the trustworthiness of the analysis). Other methods – including tables, such as matrices; graphs; charts; and networks (which connect variables through 'nodes') – can also be used to display qualitative data visually, both in the process of analysis and in the study report.

Comprehensively described by Miles and Huberman [27], these methods systematically reduce and focus the data to help make comparisons, identify patterns and themes, answer the research question, and avoid information overload of human processing capabilities. Helping to analyze single cases and facilitate cross-case analysis, the displays may be ordered, at least partially, by variables such as time. Displays may also be organized by cases; variables or concepts such as roles (e.g. patient, physician) and activities (e.g. diagnostic tests); or both. Cell entries can include, among other things, summaries, quotes and commentary.

EVALUATION OF QUALITATIVE RESEARCH

How can 'good' qualitative research be distinguished from 'poor' qualitative research? Guidelines have been developed to help evaluate qualitative research, both prospectively and retrospectively [31-33]. No consensus exists, however, on which, if any, quality criteria to apply. This is because the issue of 'quality' in qualitative research is part of a larger debate about the nature of knowledge, and its legitimate evaluation, in qualitative research [34].

In general, three positions on evaluating qualitative research can be identified:

1. Attempts to represent an underlying reality justify evaluation criteria common to quantitative and qualitative research (subtle realist position) [34].
2. Independent criteria are needed to evaluate qualitative research as a distinctive approach [35] (e.g. constructivist position, and critical change criteria [6]).
3. It is not possible to produce evaluation criteria for qualitative research, e.g. because arguably no single, coherent view of qualitative research exists (postmodern position) [36].

Evaluating these positions is beyond the scope of this book. Suffice it to say that evaluation criteria, to the extent they can be formulated, are of practical value (as indicated by their development in the first place to meet a perceived need for quality). Although these criteria vary to reflect different metatheoretical positions and methodologies (see Table 1.4), Table 4.8 suggests a basic template for critical appraisal. Organized around the pneumonic of the CRAFT of qualitative research, it suggests five evaluation criteria and strategies for meeting them.

Table 4.8. Criteria for Evaluating the Quality of Qualitative Research

Criteria	Strategy
Credibility	• Establish the credibility of the investigator
	• Demonstrate connectedness with the research, e.g. through sufficient involvement with the setting and participants
	• Report steps to enhance the rigor of the research [33]:
	1. Use multiple data sources, investigators, methods and theoretical perspectives (triangulation), appropriate to answering the study question
	2. Search for disconfirming evidence and refine the interpretation in the light of this evidence
	3. Use examples that support the descriptions and conclusions
	4. Check that the analysis flows logically and makes sense
	5. Use skeptical peer review
	6. Check that participants agree that the interpretation is defensible
	• Demonstrate consistency across the philosophical tradition, research question, methods used, and conclusions reached
Relevance: contributes to understanding	• Pose an important research question
	• Use informant checking or, ideally, actively collaborate with participants at all stages of the research
Applicability to other settings	• Fully and clearly describe the study context, methods and results, and how these influence the ability to answer the research question
Fairness	• Incorporate a range of perspectives and voices (fair dealing)
	• Be reflexive, stating your assumptions and the impact of these on the research
Trustworthiness	• Establish the credibility of the research (see above)
	• Provide an audit trail so that others may, in theory, independently review the data to corroborate the analysis

REFERENCES

[1] [Denzin N, Lincoln Y, editors. *The Sage Handbook of Qualitative Research*. Thousand Oaks: Sage Publications, 2005.

[2] Richards H, Schwartz L. Ethics of qualitative research: Are there special issues for health services research? *Fam. Pract.* 2002;19:135-9.

[3] Schwandt T. *Dictionary of Qualitative Inquiry*. 2nd Edition. Thousand Oaks: Sage Publications, 2001.

[4] Mason J. *Qualitative Researching*. London: Sage, 1996.

[5] Morse JM. What's wrong with random selection? *Qual. Health Res.* 1998;8:733-5.

[6] Patton M. *Qualitative Research and Evaluation Methods*. Thousand Oaks: Sage Publications, 2002.

[7] Becker P. Common pitfalls in published grounded theory research. *Qual. Health Res.* 1993;3:254-60.

[8] Britten N. Qualitative interviews in medical research. *BMJ* 1995;311:251-3.

[9] Markham A. *Life Online: Researching Real Experience in Virtual Space* London: Sage Publications, 1998.

[10] Couper M. Web surveys. A review of issues and approaches. *Pub. Opin. Quart* 2000;64:464-94.

[11]   Holstein J, Gubrium J. *The Active Interview. Qualitative Research Methods Series 37.* Thousand Oaks, California: Sage Publications, 1995.

[12]   Fontana A, Frey J. The interview. From neutral stance to political involvement. In: Denzin N, Lincoln Y (eds). *The Sage Handbook of Qualitative Research.* 3rd Edition. Thousand Oaks, CA: Sage Publications, 2005:695-727.

[13]   Wimpenny P, Gass J. Interviewing in phenomenology and grounded theory: is there a difference? *J. Adv. Nurs.* 2000;31:1485-92.

[14]   Geanellos R. Hermeneutic interviewing: An example of its development and use as research method. *Contemp. Nurse* 1999;8:39-45.

[15]   Greenhalgh T, Russell J, Swinglehurst D. Narrative methods in qualitative improvement research. *Qual. Saf. Health Care* 2005;14:443-9.

[16]   Spradley J. *The Ethnographic Interview.* New York: Harcourt Brace Jovanovitch, 1979.

[17]   Sorrell J, Redmond G. Interviews in qualitative nursing research: differing approaches for ethnographic and phenomenological studies. *J. Adv. Nurs.* 1995;21:1117-22.

[18]   Morgan DL. Designing Focus Group Research. In: Stewart M, Tudiver F, Bass MJ, Dunn EV, Norton PG (eds). *Tools for Primary Care Research.* Newbury Park: Sage Publications, 1992:177-93.

[19]   Grundy A, Pollon D, McGinn M. The participant as transcription: Methodological advantages of a collaborative and inclusive research practice. *Int J Qual Methods* 2003;2(2).http://www.ualberta.ca/~iiqm/backissues/2_2/pdf/grundyetal.pdf

[20]   Crichton S, Childs E. Clipping and coding audio files: A research method to enable participant voice. *Int J Qual Methods* 2005;4(3). http://www.ualberta.ca/%7Eiiqm/backissues/4_3/HTML/crichton.htm

[21]   Muller J. Narrative approaches to qualitative research in primary care. In: Crabtree B, Miller W (eds). *Doing Qualitative Research.* 2nd Edition. London: Sage Publications, 1999:221-38.

[22]   Mostyn B. The content analysis of qualitative research data: A dynamic approach. In: Brenner M, Brown J, Canter D (eds). *The Research Interview: Uses and Approaches.* New York: Academic Press, 1985.

[23]   Thomas D. A general inductive approach for analyziing qualitative evaluation data. *Am. J. Eval.* 2006;27:1-10.

[24]   Crabtree BF, Miller WL. The Analysis of Narratives from a Long Interview. In: Stewart M, Tudiver F, Bass MJ, Dunn EV, Norton PG (eds). *Tools for Primary Care Research.* Newbury Park: Sage Publications, 1992:208-20.

[25]   Glaser B. *Basics of Grounded Theory Analysis.* California: Sociology Press, 1992.

[26]   Strauss A, Corbin J. *Basics of Qualitative Research.* Thousand Oaks: Sage Publications, 1998.

[27]   Miles M, Huberman A. *Qualitative Data Analysis: A Sourcebook of New Methods.* Beverly Hills, CA: Sage, 1994.

[28]   Borkan J. Immersion/Crystallization. In: Crabtree B, Miller W (eds). *Doing Qualitative Research.* Newbury Park: Sage Publications, 1999.

[29]   Moustakas C. *Phenomenological Research Methods.* Thousand Oaks: Sage Publications, 1994.

[30]   Moustakas C. *Heuristic Research. Design, Methodology and Applications.* Newbury Park: Sage Publications, 1990.

[31]   Lincoln Y, Guba E. *Naturalistic Inquiry.* Beverly Hills, CA: Sage, 1985.

[32] Heath A. The proposal in qualitative research. *The Qualitative Report* 1997;3(1). http://www.nova.edu/ssss/QR/QR3-1/heath.html

[33] Devers K. How will we know "good" qualitative research when we see it? Beginning the dialogue in health services research. *HSR: Health Services Research* 1999;34(5 Part II):1153-88.

[34] Mays N, Pope C. Assessing quality in qualitative research. *BMJ* 2000;320:50-2.

[35] Hammersley M. *Reading Ethnographic Research*. New York: Longman, 1990.

[36] Rolfe G. Validity, trustworthiness and rigour: quality and the idea of qualitative research. *J. Adv. Nurs.* 2006;53:304-10.

Chapter 5

MINIMIZING SURVEY ERRORS

OBJECTIVES

By the time you have completed this chapter, you should be able to:

1. Describe a taxonomy of survey errors
2. Discuss the main types of survey errors
3. Suggest how to minimize the occurrence of the errors not due to measurement or processing.

PREVIEW

Error can occur at every stage of a research project, ranging from the setting of the research question to interpreting the meaning of the results. In quantitative research, error refers to the difference between a measured estimate and an unknown true value. The error may be random (or variable, i.e. due to chance), but more frequently it is systematic and produces bias. Although we can never eliminate all error, we can take steps to minimize it.

Error characterizes all study designs but this Chapter will focus on 'surveys' because their use in health research is very common. Surveys aim typically to produce cross-sectional data (Chapter 2) on a clearly delineated subject (although they may include retrospectively a longitudinal component). This chapter will present a taxonomy of total survey errors and an overview of five main types of error: sampling error, non-coverage error, non-participation error, measurement (including misclassification) error and processing error.

Approaches for dealing with the first three types of error will be discussed. Chapter 6 will elaborate on the errors of measurement and processing. The same types of error apply to other study designs in quantitative research. Although minimizing errors is a lower standard than maximizing quality, we will also learn the best methods to prevent and manage survey errors in health research.

TAXONOMY OF SURVEY ERRORS

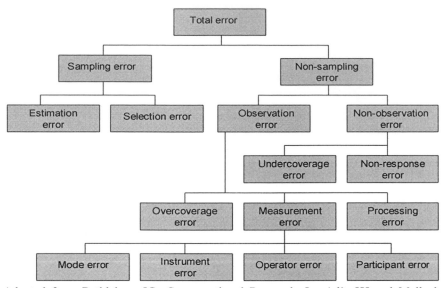

Source: Adapted from Bethlehem JG: Cross-sectional Research. In: Adèr HJ and Mellenbergh GJ. Research Methodology in the Social, Behavioural and Life Science. 1999. Sage Publications, London, pp.110-142. Or see:
http://www.blaiseusers.org/IBUCPDFS/2003/Methodological_guidelines_for.pdf

Figure 5.1. Taxonomy of Survey Errors [1].

MINIMIZING ERROR THROUGH SURVEY PLANNING AND DEVELOPMENT

Before discussing these different sources of total survey error, we need to understand the steps involved in undertaking a survey (Table 5.1). This understanding is required in order to minimize error from the outset – when setting research aims and designing the study – and to ensure collection of the information needed to assess and correct for error at the analysis stage. However, prevention is better than cure. Prevention requires the careful planning and design of research. So, it is important to record aims, hypotheses and methods before starting. This is necessary to predetermine the probability of generating a particular result. Otherwise, this probability is unknown, as the following tale illustrates:

> 'A man was wandering in a forest, and as he strolled he noticed that many trees had been used as target practice. As he came closer, he noticed that every arrow was nestled right in the bull's-eye. He marveled at the marksmanship of the archer and wondered who it might be.
> Then, in the distance, he saw a young archer taking aim at a tree. He ran over to the boy and exclaimed, "Are you the sharpshooter with all those arrows in the bull's-eyes?"
> The young boy grinned and said, "Yes, but the way I do it, it's easy. First I shoot the arrow into the tree and then I paint the bull's eye and target around it."
> Reproduced from "The Maggid Speaks" by Rabbi Paysach Kroehn with permission of the copyright holders, ArtScroll / Mesorah Publications, Ltd" [2]

Table 5.1. Process of Survey Development

	Types of data potentially needed	Reason	Example
1. Set the research aims			
2. Determine the data needed to represent the target population. Review the relevant literature.	Behavior and experience	Learn about participants' actions in the past, present or future	When do family physicians prescribe antibiotics?
	Attitudes, opinions, values	Understand the participants' perspectives on the study topic	What is your opinion of ...?
Consult with 'experts' and members of the target group	Feelings	Understand the participants' emotional response to stimuli?	How do you feel about having the surgery?
	Knowledge	Discover what the participant knows?	What is the range of services offered by your clinic?
	Sensory	Learn what is seen, heard, touched, tasted or smelled?	How would you describe your chest pain? What would you say it feels like?
	Socio-demographic and health data	Understand participants' population context and need for, and use of, services	Age, ethnicity, educational level, health status

Table 5.1 (Continued)

	Secondary data sources	Strengths	Limitations
3. Look for existing (secondary) data, which may help to meet the needs of the research	Surveys, e.g. government surveys. Key demographic sources are:	• Population-based or large samples. Data are usually low cost (money and time) to use, and may cover a wide range of topics. May be repeated and permit comparisons over time	• Need to check whether definitions used, design, and data collected meet your research needs. Changes in classification and coding limit comparisons over time
	• Population Census	• Individual enumeration, simultaneity and defined periodicity [3]. No sampling error when population-based. Detailed frames for samples and detailed data on small areas. Provide denominators (population at risk)	• Data become quickly dated. Individual topics cannot be explored in depth. Can be incomplete for some groups such as the homeless. Errors of coverage, in particular, are missed
	• Vital Statistics. Also, disease registrations and notifications	• Frequently population-based. Useful for describing and comparing frequencies of vital events and disease conditions over time and space and across different population groups	• Small number of questions because conducted mainly for administrative purposes. Subject to incomplete and delayed reporting limiting the ability to identify incident cases.
	• Special health and lifestyle surveys, e.g. Health Survey in England	• Rigorous methods typically underpin these data collections	• As above for demographic sources
	• Patients' medical records	• Valuable source of clinical data at different levels of care	• Access may require patient consent. Records tend to be incomplete and subject to classification and coding errors
	• Documentary sources, including journal articles, books and reports		

Table 5.1 (Continued)

	Types of validity	Description	How to check for this:
4. Check whether existing data (specifically the arguments made) are valid (measure what they purport to measure). Validity is needed to minimize systematic error; achieve reliability (consistency) and fulfill other criteria, such as responsiveness to change [4]	Face validity	The items appear to be valid	Expert judgment
	Content validity	The items cover all the content areas relevant to the study aims	Content Validity Index: % of items that experts rate as relevant or extremely relevant on a 4-point scale (1 = extremely irrelevant, 2 = irrelevant, 3 = relevant, and 4 = extremely irrelevant)
	Criterion-related validity	The items compare favorably with any 'gold standard' measure	Measure (a) association appropriate to measurement level of the variables; and/or (b) sensitivity and specificity
	Construct (theoretical) validity	Different items are related as expected from theory.	
	• Unidimensionality	Items in a unidimensional scale measure one underlying construct	• Perform a principal component analysis
	• Convergent validity	Items measuring similar concepts are highly correlated	• Construct a correlation matrix testing for convergent and discriminant validity together
	• Divergent validity	Items measuring different concepts are not highly correlated	

Table 5.1 (Continued)

	Types of validity	Description	How to check for this:
Reliable but not valid	Internal reliability	• Different items in a multi-item measure express the same underlying concept and so are answered in a consistent manner	Cronbach's alpha test is the most commonly used
Not valid or reliable	Inter-observer reliability	• Two or more independent observers ('raters') agree in their measurements of the same item	Cohen's Kappa test
Valid and reliable	Test-retest	• Measurements of the same items are highly associated on retest. To minimize 'reactivity' to the first test; memory effects, and change in the environment, retest 10-14 days after the first test	Calculate the correlation appropriate to the 'level of measurement' of the variables

5. Consider using or adapting an existing questionnaire, or develop a new one (using this chapter to guide us)

6. Pilot test the questionnaire, e.g. on members of our research team or on colleagues, and then on a small sample from the target population. Revise the questionnaire, as necessary

7. Collect, process and analyze (including validate, as above) our own data (see Chapter 4, and this chapter), and then report the results (Chapter 8).

Using Figure 5.1 to help structure the discussion, this chapter will now consider the main sources or types of survey errors and how to minimize them.

Sampling Error

It is efficient and economical to select a sample (population subgroup) from the sampling frame that represents our target population. However, selecting a sample introduces sampling error (or sampling variation), which is the uncertainty (rather than pure error) associated with studying a sample rather than the population. Sampling error takes two main forms: estimation error and selection error.

Estimation Error

Estimation error occurs because every sample statistic (such as a sample proportion or sample mean) is only an estimate of the true (population) value (parameter). Different samples produce different parameter estimates. This sampling variation is indicated by reporting the margin of error (confidence interval, CI) and confidence level (degree of confidence wanted) around each parameter estimate.

Usually, 95% confidence intervals are reported (see Chapter 2). For example, assume that a survey is repeated 100 times and the margin of error is ± 3% at the 95% level. If 50% give a particular response, this percentage will range from 47 to 53 (in order to include the true value) in 95 of the 100 surveys.

Selection Error

Selection error is error resulting from mistaken selection probabilities. It can result from duplicates in the sampling frame or from omissions that differ systematically from the inclusions. We should aim, therefore, to remove duplicates, or avoid omissions, in advance of the selection process. However, statistical adjustments can be made after the survey data collection. For example, we can weight the reciprocal of the number of additional times an eligible case is listed; if a case appears twice, it has double the probability of selection, so we would need to weight by one-half.

Minimizing Sampling Error

No sample can ever totally represent its source population because sampling error is unavoidable. Nevertheless, the following general strategies can be usefully adopted:

1. In general, select 'probability samples' because they permit us to estimate the sampling error and minimize this error; probability samples are the most likely to be representative of the total population. In non-probability samples, the degree to which the sample differs

Table 5.2. Types of Probability and non-Probability Sampling

Type of probability sampling	Description	Advantages	Disadvantages
Random sampling (e.g. using random number tables or the rand() function in Excel)	Each participant has the same known probability of being selected. All possible combinations are equally probable. In real sampling situations, all sampling is without replacement	Permits 'statistical inference'; i.e. on the basis of probability theory, it allows generalizations from the sample to a target population of which it is representative	Can be costly and difficult to do
Stratified random sampling	Individuals are selected randomly in *each* stratum (e.g. males and females) into which the sampling frame has been divided for analysis. Strata sample sizes may be proportional or not to the population sizes in the strata	Can improve the efficiency of the sample (i.e. gain increased accuracy for the same cost), especially in strata that vary markedly in size.	As above. Disproportionate stratification can produce estimators that are less precise than those obtained through a random sample of the same size
Cluster sampling	'Natural' groupings (e.g. schools or geographic areas) or 'clusters' become the unit that is sampled	Reduces costs associated with dispersed populations	Less statistically efficient, if the clusters are homogenous, than simple random sampling
• Single stage cluster design	Sampling occurs once: Select one or more clusters (e.g. randomly), then every unit in the cluster(s)	Useful when no sampling list is available for units within clusters	Produces more error than does a simple random sample for a given sample size. This error is reduced if the clusters are similar, but high if the clusters are different
• Multistage sampling	Sampling occurs ≥ 2 times; e.g. select clusters (e.g. districts) and then sample units (e.g. households) within these clusters. Where units vary in size, select the units from a stratified sample or sample with a probability proportional to unit size	Sampling with a probability proportional to size ensures a proportionately greater likelihood of selecting the sampling units with the largest populations	Makes the analysis more complicated than for simple random sampling
Systematic sampling	The first participant is selected randomly. Then, every nth (e.g. 5th) participant is selected	Simpler than random sampling for large samples. Permits even spread.	Bias can occur if the list sampled from (e.g. surnames) has been ordered or has a cyclical characteristic (non-random)

Table 5.2 (Continued)

Type of probability sampling	Description	Advantages	Disadvantages
Convenience (availability) sampling	Participants (e.g. volunteers) are selected because they are accessible	Can generate large numbers of participants, survey rare population groups, and usefully identify a range of perspectives	Often not representative of the target population
Quota sampling (model-based sampling)	Participants are selected non-randomly within strata to get a specified composition (e.g. two-thirds female, one-third male)	Can produce valuable insights. Is cheap, convenient and requires no sampling frame	May be unrepresentative and biased. No valid estimate of the risk of errors
Judgment sampling (also known as purposive sampling; lesson 4)	Particular participants are selected intentionally on the basis of the investigator's judgment or discretion	Can be used to represent the phenomenon of interest	As above

Table 5.3. Margins of Error for Different Sample Sizes and Levels of Confidence

Margin of error %*	Sample size (for percents)*	
	95% level of confidence	99% level of confidence
2	2144	3435
3	1014	1688
4	583	986
5	377	643
6	264	451
7	195	333
10	96	165
14	49	85

* Assumes conservatively that for each question the percentage giving a particular response is 50%; this yields the largest sample size

from the population is unknown. Table 5.2 describes and evaluates different types of probability and non-probability samples [5].

2. Increase the sample size, but up to a point: diminishing returns (Table 5.3) require a trade-off between costs and the precision of estimates. Also, too large a sample may suggest statistically significant differences that do not exist (type 1 error) or are clinically unimportant. Small samples can suggest that clinically important differences do not exist when they really do (type 2 error).
3. Adjust selection probabilities, e.g. through careful investigation of the sampling frame and strategies such as stratified random sampling.
4. Carefully check the sampling frame to avoid omissions and duplicates

NON-SAMPLING ERROR

Even with complete enumeration of the target population, non-sampling error can occur. This error, which is not due to the sampling method and sample size, comprises non-observation error and observation error.

Non-Observation Error

Non-observation error occurs when all or some of the measurements intended cannot be made on some part of the target population or sample. This error comprises non-coverage error and non-response error. Table 5.4 describes both types of error, their causes and how to manage them.

Non-response error tends to be associated with low response rates (low participation rates); that is, low proportions of all eligible units (e.g. individuals or households) that complete the questionnaire or other data collection instrument [6]. Most researchers attempt

Table 5.4. Non-Observation Errors

Type	Description	Cause	Solution
Under-coverage	Omission of some cases that are not part of the intended target population (eligibles)	List of cases is incomplete, out of date, or both	• Clearly define the target population in advance • Use the most complete and current list available. • Consider using multiple lists • Make post-survey adjustments, such as weighting
		Clustering (e.g. the frame lists households, but you wish to sample a household member)	• Assign to each selected participant a weight proportional to the number of other eligible members in her or his (household) grouping
Non-participation error	Participants differ from non-participants (unit non-participation)	Some participants are not contactable	• Vary the contact pattern, e.g. phone at different times • Consider different modes of contact, e.g. phone and post • Consider whether the reason for the non-contact is random or systematic, e.g. poor people may be less likely to have a telephone and may change their address more often than other people • Seek to obtain information (e.g. gender) about these non-participants (and non-contactable ones) so that an assessment can be made as to whether they differ from the participants on selected variables
		Some designated participants are incapable of taking part	
		Some participants refuse to take part (non-cooperation)	• Use strategies to increase participation rates (Figure 5.2) • Post-survey adjustments: • Weight the data for non-response • Model the non-response • Check whether a low response rate necessarily produces bias

Table 5.4 (Continued)

Type	Description	Cause	Solution
		Some participants drop out (have moved or died)	• Forward tracing: at the initial interview, ask participants for contact details of someone who will know how to reach them if they change their address
			• Contact participants between measurements and use change of address notifications that the Post Office provides when it has been told of the movement
	Participants who answer certain questions differ from those who do not (item non-participation)	'Don't know' responses	• Discourage these responses. Use probes delivered by trained interviewers (see Table 6.8)
		Questions skipped owing by participants or interviewer owing to measurement error	• Correct navigational errors in advance (see Table 6.4). Handle missing data appropriately, e.g. by imputing values for the missing data
		Refusals	• Desensitize questions, e.g. by using income categories as response options

to maximize response rates (although high response rates do not necessarily reduce non-response error [7]). The effectiveness of strategies for minimizing the non-response error is likely to depend on the type of participants targeted.

Figure 5.2 quantifies estimates of the effectiveness of different strategies for minimizing non-response error during recruitment in surveys with the public. However, a recent systematic review of randomized trials in health research [8] questions the value of incentives in maximizing responses to postal questionnaires. The review confirms the high importance of repeat mailing strategies and telephone reminders.

Strategy	No of trials (No of participants)	Odds ratio (95% CI)	P value for heterogeneity
Incentives			
Monetary incentive v no incentive	49 (46 474)	2.02 (1.79 to 2.27)	<0.00001
Incentive with questionnaire v incentive on return	10 (13 713)	1.71 (1.29 to 2.26)	<0.00001
Non-monetary incentive v no incentive	45 (44 708)	1.19 (1.11 to 1.28)	<0.00001
Length			
Shorter v longer questionnaire	40 (40 669)	1.86 (1.55 to 2.24)	<0.00001
Appearance			
Brown envelope v white	2 (5311)	1.52 (0.67 to 3.44)	<0.00001
Coloured ink v standard	1 (3540)	1.39 (1.16 to 1.67)	
Folder or booklet v stapled pages	2 (1845)	1.17 (0.94 to 1.45)	
More personalised v less personalised	38 (39 210)	1.16 (1.06 to 1.28)	<0.00001
Identifying feature on return v none	7 (4014)	1.08 (0.78 to 1.51)	<0.001
Coloured questionnaire v white	8 (14 797)	1.06 (0.99 to 1.14)	
Delivery			
Recorded delivery v standard	6 (2127)	2.21 (1.51 to 3.25)	<0.01
Stamped returned envelope v business reply or franked	14 (38 259)	1.26 (1.13 to 1.41)	<0.00001
Questionnaire sent to work address v home address	2 (1140)	1.16 (0.89 to 1.52)	
First class outward mailing v other class	1 (7370)	1.12 (1.02 to 1.23)	
Pre-paid return envelope v not pre-paid	4 (4094)	1.09 (0.71 to 1.68)	<0.00001
Stamped outward envelope v franked	6 (13 964)	0.95 (0.88 to 1.03)	
Commemorative stamp v ordinary stamp	4 (5238)	0.92 (0.78 to 1.09)	
Contact			
Precontact v no precontact	28 (28 793)	1.54 (1.24 to 1.92)	<0.00001
Follow up v no follow up	12 (16 740)	1.44 (1.22 to 1.70)	<0.0001
Postal follow up including questionnaire v postal follow up excluding questionnaire	6 (6310)	1.41 (1.02 to 1.94)	<0.00001
Mention of follow up contact v none	6 (6553)	1.04 (0.91 to 1.18)	
Precontact by telephone v post	2 (1375)	0.90 (0.70 to 1.16)	
Content			
More interesting v less interesting questionnaire	2 (2151)	2.44 (1.99 to 3.01)	
User friendly questionnaire v standard	1 (3540)	1.46 (1.21 to 1.75)	
Factual questions only v factual and attitudinal	1 (1280)	1.34 (1.01 to 1.77)	
More relevant questions first v other items first	1 (5817)	1.23 (1.10 to 1.37)	
Demographic items first v other items first	2 (1040)	1.04 (0.81 to 1.34)	
'Don't know' boxes included v not included	1 (1360)	1.03 (0.82 to 1.29)	
Sensitive question included v no sensitive question	6 (19 851)	0.92 (0.87 to 0.98)	
Most general question first v last	1 (2000)	0.80 (0.67 to 0.96)	
Origin			
University sponsorship or as source v other organisation	13 (20 428)	1.31 (1.11 to 1.54)	<0.00001
Sent by more senior or well known person v less senior or less well known	4 (2584)	1.13 (0.95 to 1.35)	
Ethnically unidentifiable/white name v other name	2 (1800)	1.11 (0.91 to 1.36)	
Communication			
Explanation for not participating requested v not requested	1 (1240)	1.32 (1.05 to 1.66)	
Appeal stresses benefit to respondent v other	6 (9332)	1.06 (0.92 to 1.22)	
Appeal stresses benefit to sponsor v other	7 (9708)	1.01 (0.86 to 1.19)	<0.05
Appeal stresses benefit to society v other	8 (10 088)	1.00 (0.84 to 1.20)	<0.01
Response deadline given v no deadline	4 (4340)	1.00 (0.84 to 1.20)	<0.05
Instructions given v not given	1 (2000)	0.89 (0.74 to 1.06)	
Choice to opt out from study given v none	3 (3045)	0.76 (0.65 to 0.89)	

0.1 0.2 0.5 1 2 3 4 5

Response lower with first category · Response higher with first category

Odds ratio

Source: *BMJ* 2002; 324: 1183. Reproduced with permission from the BMJ Publishing Group.

Figure 5.2. How to Minimize Non-Participation Error during Recruitment [9].

Observation Error

During the data collection, observation error comprises overcoverage error, measurement error and processing error. Overcoverage error refers to including some cases that are not part of the target population (ineligibles). The amount of bias this produces depends on how many such cases are selected and the extent to which they differ from eligible cases. Try to screen for, and discard, ineligibles, although reducing the number of ineligibles may also reduce the number of eligibles (increase under-coverage).

Errors of Measurement and Processing

Measurement error [10] is error resulting from uncertainty or variation between measurements. This type of error is inevitable but can be minimized, for example by posing questions that are answerable, valid, reliable and useful. In turn, processing error denotes error in data processing and analysis. Table 5.5 uses the example of blood pressure measurement to illustrate sources of error in measurement and processing.

Table 5.5. Sources of Error of Measurement and Processing

Sources	Definition	Example of blood pressure measurement
Mode error	Wrong instrument is used.	Use of digital rather than manometric type of blood pressure meter
Instrument error	Difference between the true value and the value indicated by the instrument.	The mercury sphygmomanometer has lost some mercury
Operator error	Error in how the instrument is administered.	The clinician has a hearing or sight deficit
Participant error (response error)	Error in responding to the instrument	The patient is anxious about the measurement (Hawthorne effect)
Processing error, e.g. confounding	Error in processing (recording and managing) the data and analyzing the results	No steps are taken to avoid confounding

REFERENCES

[1] Bethlehem, JG. Cross-sectional research. In: Ader H, Mellenbergh G (eds). *Research Methodology in the Social, Behavioural and Life Sciences*. London: Sage Publications, 1999:110-42.

[2] Kroehn PR. *The Maggid Speaks*. Brooklyn: NY: ArtScroll / Mesorah Publications, Ltd, 1987.

[3] Shryock H, Siegel J and associates. *The Methods and Materials of Demography*. Washington DC: US Bureau of the Census, 1980.

[4] Viswanathan M. *Measurement Error and Research Design*. Thousand Oaks, CA: Sage, 2005.

[5] Kish L. *Survey Sampling*. New York: John Wiley and Sons, 1995.

[6]   Weisberg H. *The Total Survey Error Approach*. Chicago: University of Chicago Press, 2005.

[7]   Krosnick J. Survey research. *Ann Rev Psychol* 1999;50:537-67.

[8]   Nakash R, Hutton J, Jorstad-Stein E, Gates S, Lamb S. Maximising response to postal questionnaires - A systematic review of randomised trials in health research. *BMC Med Res Method* 2006.

[9]   Edwards P, Roberts I, Clarke M, DiGuiseppi S, Wentz R, Kwan I. Increasing responses rates to postal questionnaires: systematic review. *BMJ* 2002;324:1183-91.

[10] Biemer P, Groves R, Lyberg L, Mathiowetz N, Sudman S (eds). *Measurement Error in Surveys*. New York: John Wiley and Sons, Inc, 1991.

Chapter 6

MEASUREMENT ERRORS AND PROCESSING ERRORS IN SURVEY RESEARCH

OBJECTIVES

By the time you have completed this chapter, you should be able to:

1. Discuss the main types of errors of measurement and processing respectively
2. Suggest how to minimize the occurrence of these errors

PREVIEW

This chapter elaborates on the non-sampling observation errors of measurement and processing respectively. Each of these types of error will be described. Concurrent consideration of how to minimize them (e.g. by taking advantage of the benefits of different methods) helps to balance the discussion. As an extension of the preceding chapter, the spotlight will again be on the occurrence of errors in survey research, while recognizing that these also characterize other quantitative study designs.

Focusing on interviews and self-complete questionnaires, this chapter will first look at how to ask sensible questions sensibly through understanding and managing the different types of measurement error. Mode error can occur when questions are inappropriately administered via self-completion rather than interview, or *vice versa*; and Table 4.4 summarized some insights into this issue. However, we will focus here on three other types of measurement error: instrument error, participant error and, as a form of operator error, interviewer error (as introduced at the end of Chapter 5). A few of the tables apply only to self-complete questionnaires, but most are relevant to self-complete questionnaires and interviews.

Secondly, we will consider how to make sensible use of the data collected during health survey research. This involves minimizing processing errors by appropriately preparing and analyzing the data collected, and interpreting basic statistics that have been produced through the process of data analysis.

Instrument Error

The following discussion focuses on instrument error, interviewer (operator) error and participant error. With regard to instrument error, Table 6.1 refers to specific question (item) errors that should be avoided in interviews and self-complete questionnaires. We will then focus on errors in question sequencing (Tables 6.2) before reviewing formatting errors that are important to minimize (Table 6.3) [1 2].

Table 6.1. Question Wording Errors

Error	Reason	Example
Unclear (including ambiguous) questions for the target audience	Participants might not understand the question or vary in their understanding	How many members are there in your family?
Leading questions (and loaded words) implying that a particular answer is expected or socially desirable	Lack of neutrality can produce an acquiescence bias (Table 6.7)	Do you prefer to be examined by a doctor of your own sex?
Double-barreled questions (posing two questions in one)	Participants may be answering only one question but which one may be unclear	Have you suffered from headaches or nausea recently?
Double-negative questions	These questions invite an ambiguous response	Are you not required to provide an annual health check?
Long questions (more than, say, 20 words)	These questions are difficult to follow and remember, which can make responses difficult	In the last 12 months, has your child's wheezing ever been severe enough to limit her/his speech to only one or two words at a time between breaths?
Non-gender neutral pronouns despite referring to no specific gender	These can be perceived to devalue the unnamed gender	When you see the nurse, does she usually weigh you?
'Why' questions may be erroneous	A cause-effect relationship may not exist. Participants may respond defensively to these and future questions	Instead of: why did you delay getting a mammogram? Ask: what discouraged you from getting a mammogram?
Questions with low discriminatory power	Almost everyone will provide the same answer	How satisfied are you with your usual doctor?
Irrelevant and redundant questions (except to check intra-respondent reliability)	These questions waste time and can alienate respondents	Personal details that are unimportant
General questions	The meaning intended can be unclear	Did you see a physician last year?
Questions whose answers are likely to change rapidly	Associated with low test-retest reliability	How welcoming are the receptionists in your practice?
Mixing elliptical (shortened) and non-elliptical questions	These questions can shift response patterns and introduce bias	How come? Vs How did you reach this decision?
Response options that are not mutually exclusive	These options can produce invalid responses	Are you aged ≤ 65 or ≥ 65?
Response options that are not mutually exhaustive	Can produce invalid responses	Are you aged < 65 or > 65?

Table 6.1 (Continued)

Error	Reason	Example
Too many response options	Some may be redundant	Detailed breakdown of marital status may be unnecessary
Scale point proliferation	Can annoy or confuse participants	9-point Likert scale (see Table 6.5)
Tag questions (posing two questions, one after the other)	Participants may rush an answer to the first question because they do not want to forget the second question	How would you describe your receptionist? How would you describe the practice manager?"
Questions that are over-precise, are too demanding, or that participants cannot answer	These frustrate participants and invite invalid responses or high levels of non-response	Rank these 20 factors in order of importance.

Table 6.2. Question Sequencing Errors

Placement	Errors	Solution	Rationale
Opening questions	Sensitive or threatening questions Participants vary in their willingness to write responses	• Start with easy to answer, non-threatening and relevant questions. This helps to motivate candid, interested responses, while minimizing question refusals. Ice-breaker questions can help to establish rapport in interviews	• Ice-breaker questions permit participants to introduce themselves. This involves them early, helps them to relax, and provides valuable contextual information
Middle questions	Questions of low relevance Questions that do not flow logically Uninteresting questions	• Ask the questions most relevant to the study aims. Place any difficult questions here • Group questions on each common topic, but scattering neutral questions can help to buffer the context effects of items that may influence one another. Intersperse fact-based questions • Usually ask about the present before the past or future • Mix the direction of closed questions to avoid participants giving the same response	• It is important to ask key questions before participants tire • The logical flow of questions, and interspersal of fact-based questions, helps to prevent participants disengaging. • It is usually easiest to talk about the present before the past or future
Closing questions	Questions that leave participants feeling low Difficult questions Failure to allow participants to add additional information	• End on a positive note, that 'cools' down the interview or the questionnaire self-administration. • Make questions easy to answer • Place demographic questions at the end • Check for participants' own questions	• It is necessary to allow time to establish rapport and to avoid termination of the interview before key information is collected

Once we have selected or developed our questions, we need to consider how best to sequence them in our questionnaire, since the question order and resultant positioning may influence the responses given. Table 6.2 conceptualizes errors in question sequencing in terms of mistiming questions within questionnaires. These issues apply mainly to interviews because respondents to self-complete questionnaires may read all the questions before answering, and give more considered responses.

Various aspects of the formatting and physical appearance of self-complete questionnaires can influence the willingness and ability of people to participate and, in turn, can affect the survey response rate, the amount of missing data on particular questions and the quality of responses to the questions that participants answer. The format of interview schedules can also contribute to interviewer error. Table 6.3 therefore suggests and explains ways to avoid different formatting errors.

Table 6.3. Questionnaire Format

Error	Solution	Rationale
Unbound questionnaires	Use booklets On a front cover state the survey title, the organization running the survey and an identification number	• Help not to lose pages • Maximize participation rates • Help the participant, interviewer and data processor move through the questionnaire • Help the participant stay alert and not provide a response that is 'good enough' but not optimal • Prevent accidentally skipping questions to ask and answer • Prevent incorrect recording of answers by interviewers • Motivate completion of the questionnaire • Make the questionnaire easier to process
Complex, unclear formats	Use a large, clear typeface Use white paper or a light tint to increase legibility Provide instructions at the point where they are needed Order questions logically Seek to avoid splitting questions across two pages	

Table 6.3 (Continued)

Error	Solution
	Use a consistent question format
	List response choices in a single column (except for rating scales), with boxes consistently on the left or right
	Use mechanical devices such as arrows and boxes (i.e. make question sequences easy to follow)
	Number the questions and pages of the questionnaire
Poor use of space and crowding questions	Put more space between questions than between questions and answers
	Provide enough space to record answers
	Avoid putting lines for responses to open questions
Overlong questionnaires	Choose an appropriate questionnaire length (2 to 4 pages for surveys that have low salience to the population).Use double-sided printing
Monotonous presentations	Print any personalized cover letter on letterhead stationery; the lead researcher should sign the letter in blue)
Separate interviewer instructions	Place clear instructions (and probes), possibly in italics, alongside the questions to which they pertain

PARTICIPANT ERROR

Next we will focus on how the limitations or misuse of otherwise appropriate questions can produce errors that participants make. Table 4.4 compared advantages and disadvantages of self-complete questionnaires and interviews in qualitative research, but also has relevance here. Table 6.4 describes and evaluates the open and closed formats of questions associated with both of these methods of questionnaire administration in survey research. Although these question formats each have advantages, their limitations – even when used in ways that do not constitute instrument error or interviewer error – can produce error in how participants cognitively process and respond to questions.

Table 6.5 critiques different closed question formats (ordered and unordered categories) for the measurement of participant attitudes. These formats are especially common in self-complete questionnaires but they can also be used in interviews. For a discussion of open question formats, see Chapter 4.

Participant error can also result from how questionnaires are structured [3] Table 6.6 considers funnel, pyramid and diamond structures. Each of these structures has limitations, which are intensified by any design, or operator, failure to apply the most appropriate structure in a given situation. Consistent with the guidance in Table 6.2 on question sequencing errors, most questionnaires follow a funnel structure [4]. However, Table 6.6 indicates when other design structures may or may not be more appropriate. As noted above, only interviews can control sequencing effects because participants may read ahead in self-complete questionnaires, negating any intended effect of question sequencing.

Table 6.4. Question Formats

Type	Description	Advantages	Disadvantages
Open (free response and text open) questions	Cannot be answered with a predetermined response option (single word or short phrase). Beyond this restriction, participants can respond as they choose in text	• In development stages and pilot studies they can produce appropriate response categories • Easy to ask • Stimulate free thought • Allow participants to respond freely, permitting depth and breadth of response as well as quotable material • Indicate areas for further questioning, and possible response categories • Interest participants	• Can be difficult and time-consuming to answer and analyze • May produce much irrelevant detail • Subject to interviewer variance • Can lead to loss of control of the interview
Partially closed questions	Includes numeric open end, and questions offering some responses but permitting participants to produce their own; e.g. 'other, please describe _____'	• Permit the inclusion of important reasons not thought of by the investigator(s) • Ensure the response set is exhaustive	• Tend not to discourage participants from selecting from the closed responses given • As below
Closed questions	Require participants to select the best answer from a fixed set of predetermined response options	• Permit codes next to closed responses • Can be memory cues or suggest latent issues • Quickly generate precise, concise, standardized and relevant data that are usually easy to analyze • Require little skill to administer in interviews; keep control of the conversation	• Produce thin data • Easy to answer without adequate thought • May lead participants who cannot consider all the alternatives at once to select the first plausible response or the last response • May frustrate participants who disagree with the response options or find them uninteresting • Lose spontaneity and expressiveness • Can miss key ideas and detail • Have potential for bias from the wording of the response categories

Table 6.5. Closed Response Formats for Attitude Measurement

Type	Definition	Example	Advantages	Disadvantages
Likert-type scale	Unidimensional scale rating individual items from strongly disagree to strongly agree	Accessibility to the clinic Strongly disagree / Disagree / Neutral / Agree / Strongly agree Item 1 ☐ ☐ ☐ ☐ ☐ Item 2 ☐ ☐ ☐ ☐ ☐	• Can measure most attitudes • Familiar to many participants • Easy to read and answer • Odd number of response options permits a middle or neutral position	• Can be difficult to decide which items 'go together' and how best to combine them • Prone to ceiling effects (clustering of responses at ends of scale) that may conceal true variation • Prone to bias toward positive evaluations
Pictorial scale	Unidimensional scale depicting pictorially its response categories	How do you feel about visiting the doctor? 	• Entertaining. • Suited to participants with low literacy, e.g. very young; cognitively impaired; and poorly educated	• May be ambiguous • Cannot make fine distinctions

Table 6.5 (Continued)

Type	Definition	Example	Advantages	Disadvantages
Visual analogue scale	Unidimensional continuous scale depicted on a line, usually 10 cm, between two anchor statements. Participants mark the line to respond. Investigator measures the distance to the mark	Completely dissatisfied 0 cm / Completely satisfied 10 cm	• Permits a continuous assessment • Prevents participants from knowing what score they give • Useful for participants with limited verbal skills and for comparing changes within participants	• Expects participants to have the cognitive ability to express experience in analogue form and understand proportionality • Less time and cost efficient for investigator than are numeric and verbal scales
Rank list	Unidimensional scale comprising items that participants are required to rank	Rank the following in order of importance: Item 1 ☐ Item 2 ☐ Item 3 ☐ Item 4 ☐ Rank Values must be between 1 and 4	• Produces excellent discrimination among responses	• Requires short list to rank but still tends to be more difficult and to take longer to complete than rating scales • Does not reveal any baseline or by how much one item is preferred over another • Prone to participant error

Table 6.5 (Continued)

Type	Definition	Example	Advantages	Disadvantages
Semantic differential scales	Rate attitudes on a number of bipolar adjectival scales of opposite responses	Shared decision-making Unimportant ▢ ▢ ▢ ▢ ▢ ▢ Important Impractical ▢ ▢ ▢ ▢ ▢ ▢ Practical	• Suited to measuring attitudes and feelings simply • Offers an alternative to the counterintuitive Likert approach of negating constructs to avoid acquiescence bias	• Can be difficult to define true opposites • Assumes that the adjectives chosen mean the same to everyone • Imposes higher cognitive demand on participants than do Likert scales • May result in the answer to the first item producing an 'anchor' against which participants adjust their ratings of subsequent items • May lead participants to answer a series of closed questions in the same way (response set bias) • Usual problems of rating scales, such as acquiescence bias, and social desirability bias

Table 6.6. Questionnaire Structure

Structure	Description	Rationale	Risk of participant error
Funnel	Begins with broad, open questions and narrows the scope of questions to closed, specific questions	• Gets participants talking and aids rapport building. • Participants can help to define and respond, with minimum interviewer input and without delay, to complex issues they may feel passionately about	• Participants may lack ideas about the topic, or need more interviewer input, at the beginning of the interview
Pyramid	Begins with narrow, closed and specific questions before working toward open questions	• Eases participants into a generalized discussion of issues that they may be hesitant to address, before posing the most challenging questions • Ensures consideration of some points before evaluations are made. News reporters commonly use this approach	• Can frustrate participants who need to express their ideas without early restraint • Detailed early questions may focus on issues unimportant to participants • May feel threatening to participants who have no time to relax
Diamond	Starts with closed, specific questions, moves toward open questions, and ends with closed questions that focus on the participant's specific requirements	• Variety provided may help to sustain the participant's interest and attention	• As for the pyramid structure • Can unsettle participants by returning to closed questions • Time consuming and hence potentially tiring

Lastly, participants' awareness of being 'observed' can cause them to misperceive demand characteristics of the research; that is, the study conditions may appear to participants to demand from them a certain kind of response to tasks posed. This perception can lead participants to change their response behavior (Hawthorne effect), for example by misreporting information, intentionally or unintentionally, in a systematic manner. The result is various types of participant bias as summarized in Table 6.7.

INTERVIEWER ERROR

We will now look at the operator errors associated with interviewing and what can be done to minimize their occurrence and severity. We will start by summarizing interviewing styles (Table 6.8) [5 6], noting how each style can produce interviewer errors, e.g. in the questions that interviewers pose.

Table 6.7. Participant Bias

Bias	Tendency of participants to:	Remedy
Apathy bias	Take little or no care in answering questions	• Make the survey as short, interesting and easy to answer as possible
Auspices or sponsorship bias	Report what they think the sponsor wants to hear	• Use independent groups to conduct the survey • Avoid disclosing the sponsor
Acquiescence bias	Agree with the items presented to them	• Usc balanced questions • Express items in a mixture of positive and negative ways
Extremity bias	Give or avoid extreme responses	• Use open questions that avoid extreme categories
Negation bias	Disagree with the items presented to them	• Use open questions or a mixture of positively and negatively worded items
Prestige bias	Respond in a way that makes them feel good	• Seek to minimize the prestige associated with question wording. • Maximize anonymity; e.g. prefer self-complete questionnaires to interviews
Recall bias	Recall past events inaccurately or incompletely	• Minimize the recall period. • Give increased time, e.g. ask longer questions. • Provide memory cues; e.g. relate to landmark events or reconstruct past processes
Social desirability bias	To report what they believe is socially acceptable or politically correct	• Include reasonable excuses ('forgiving words') • Administer self-complete surveys • Favor open and longer questions • Use familiar words • Consider loading questions (so that they lead toward the view deemed socially undesirable) • Embed an undesirable option among other options to reduce its salience • Encourage participants to believe that false responses can be detected

Participants sometimes give responses that are incomplete, unclear or not appropriately responsive. Interviews, unlike self-complete questionnaires, offer an opportunity to probe in order to elicit additional information, and prompt (as a not necessarily linguistic device) to facilitate the interview flow. Probes and prompts may be planned or informal [8]. Table 6.9 summarizes potential errors associated with their use or not, and how to use them appropriately to prevent making errors.

Table 6.8. Interviewing Style

Style	Description	Risk of error	Solution
Rapport building approach	Develops a good professional relationship with participants	Overly personalizing the interviews	• Seek equanimity as a middle ground between empathy and detachment [7]
Motivational approach	Motivates participants, through building commitment, to optimize rather than to respond in a minimally acceptable manner	As above. Motivation is not well understood	• Incorporate other interviewing styles
Standardized approach	Asks the same questions in the same way of all participants	Reduced ability to clarify ambiguities in question wording	• Focus on the clarity of questions with standardized wording • Use a conversational approach
Conversational (flexible) approach	Permits the interviewer to depart from standardized wording to clarify the intended meaning of questions	Increased risk of interviewer errors, such as skip errors and recording errors. Findings may lack reliability if participants receive different stimuli	• Provide proper training, supervision and monitoring

Table 6.9. Probes and Prompts

Potential errors	Solutions	Example
Probes and prompts may result in some participants receiving different stimuli from others	Standardized interviewing	
Failure to probe or prompt Incorrect use: • Directive • Non-neutral • Ineffective, e.g. can be answered 'yes' or 'no'	Conversational interviewing	
	• Use of neutral and non-directive probes, e.g. in response to 'don't knows'	
	Expanding	Tell me more about…
	Clarifying	Help me to understand…
	Justifying	Can you explain…?
	Consequential	What is the result of…?
	Contrast	What is the difference between…?

Table 6.9 (Continued)

Potential errors	Solutions	Example
	• Appropriate use of prompts	
	Repeat the question or explain in other words	
	Echo prompt (repeat the particiapnt's last word)	
	Reflective summary of what participant has just said)	
	Recapitulation (summarize what the participant said earlier)	
	Silence (permissive pause)	
	Attentive lean (head nod)	
	Affirmative noise (e.g. uh huh)	

Lastly, Table 6.10 takes the form of a checklist, which summarizes various steps that can be taken before, during and after interviews in order to reduce the risk of interviewer error.

Table 6.10. Steps to minimize interviewer error

Before the interview	• Become familiar with the nature and requirements of the interview; pre-test the interview instrument, in a non-threatening environment, on experts and persons similar to the participants
	• Explain to potential participants the purpose and conditions of the interview, including confidentiality and audiotaping
	• Schedule sufficient time for the interview
	• Remind participants of their interview 1 to 2 days beforehand
	• Dress and groom appropriately for the interview
	• Arrive on time
	• Prepare and bring the necessary equipment (a good audiorecorder with a labeled tape ready to record; spare tapes wound back, spare batteries, an extension lead, paper and pens)
At the interview	• Attempt to choose a private and quiet setting, free from outside interruptions or distractions
	• Introduce the interview. Review its purpose, use of results, any risks, and the rights of participants. Do not say too much early on as this can lead participants to say what they think we want to hear.
	• Check acceptance before collecting any data (including consent to audiotape)
	• Remind participants that they can end the interview at any time
	• Anticipate problems (e.g. make notes in case the audiorecorder fails)
	• Position the audiorecorder between the interviewer and the participant. Test it immediately before the interview begins

Table 6.10 (Continued)

	• Seek to develop a rapport with, and the trust of, the participant
	• Emphasize the importance of what the participant thinks
	• Communicate clearly in the participant's terms
	• Relax. Be friendly, respectful and yet candid. Show interest in what the participant says
	• Let the participant speak most
	• Sequence logically the questions and larger topic areas
	• Give the participant time to think; be comfortable with silence: extended silences can indicate a problem
	• Listen carefully. Don't interrupt or finishes sentences for the participant
	• Stay neutral: Try to bracket out our own views and not judge the participant or appear shocked by what we hear or see
	• Give some control to the participant but protect the orderliness and integrity of the interview
	• Restrict the interview to a maximum of 60 to 90 minutes
	• End on a positive note and thank the participant
	• Probe and persist to obtain politely the detail needed. Keep the participant focused on answering balanced questions
	• Observe non-verbal behavior and the setting
	• Record impressions but balance eye contact with looking away
End of the interview	• Summarize the main points to check our own understanding
Immediately after the interview	• Test the audiotape and write up our notes

PROCESSING ERROR

Numerous errors can occur in processing the data collected. These include errors in data handling (e.g. data coding, data entry and data transfer), in data analysis, in data documentation and in data interpretation. The most important of these errors are described below. Good planning can avoid or minimize many of them but steps during the data analysis are also needed to manage the errors.

Confounding

To understand confounding, consider a relationship between an exposure and an outcome. Confounding takes place when a third variable (a 'confounder') provides an alternative explanation for this relationship. A confounder is related to, and may be a cause of, both the outcome and the exposure. However, it cannot be an effect of either and it is unequally distributed between those with the exposure and those without it (Figure 6.1). For example, we might falsely attribute high blood pressure to diet rather than to anxiety associated with both the diet and raised blood pressure.

As a result, the effect of the exposure cannot be distinguished from the effect of the confounder. This is common in observational studies because of non-randomized allocation to the study groups. Failure to consider, and account for, the effect of the confounder can lead to measuring incorrectly the effect of the exposure of interest. Note that factors mediating the relationship between the exposure and outcome of interest (intermediate variables) are not confounders.

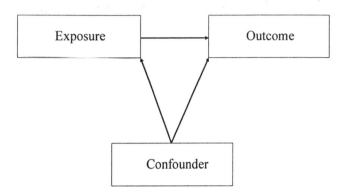

Figure 6.1. A Simple Model of Confounding

To minimize confounding error:

1. Conduct the study in populations in which the exposure of interest and potential confounders are not strongly associated with each other.
2. Include only participants who are similar in relation to the confounder; for example, in the figure above, include only patients who are not anxious.
3. Collect data on known or potential confounders, which can be used to adjust statistically for these variables at the analysis stage.

We will now consider how to avoid or remedy a range of problems, which have the potential to introduce error, by preparing and analyzing our data appropriately (Table 6.11) [9 10].

Table 6.11. How to Avoid Errors through Data Preparation and Analysis

Problem	Remedy at the data analysis stage
Categorical variables tend to convey the least information about participants, and permit use of the least powerful statistical tests	• Create dichotomous variables (because these can be treated as continuous variables) from other categorical (nominal or ordinal) variables. (Nominal level variables name variables (e.g. religions) without any rank ordering. Ordinal level variables rank variables (e.g. from high to low) but cannot specify the size of numerical differences. Interval level (continuous) variables enumerate values (e.g. years of age) that are numerically meaningful, revealing the size of differences between them) • Treat ordinal data (e.g. Likert scales) as if they are interval data if an underlying metric can be assumed • Convert grouped numerical variables to the interval level, if we believe that participants are evenly distributed within each group • Use a statistical method appropriate to the use of nominal or ordinal variables

Table 6.11 (Continued)

Problem	Remedy at the data analysis stage
There is a need to avoid or detect errors in data entry	• Use professionals for data entry • Use double entry methods • Use a data entry template • Scan frequency counts for errors
The variables needed are unavailable	• Compute new variables that combine information from existing variables, or modify a single variable (e.g. divide annual visits by 12 to derive monthly visits)
There are too many variables	• Reduce the number of variables, e.g. into single composite measures
Some variables fail to discriminate between participants (e.g. 90% of patients might report high satisfaction with their practice)	• Do not use the variable • Use the non-discriminating variable with other variables • When there are 2 or 3 non-discriminating categories, recode them to focus on the variation between them
The large number of categories makes tables and figures difficult to read. The categories with few cases are unreliable	• Use statistical methods that can handle such data • Reduce the number of categories through recoding: *Substantive recoding*: combines the categories that seem to belong together whereas *distributional recoding* combines categories into a reduced number of equal size
Categories are arranged with no logical order; this can make tables difficult to read, and conceal an ordinal level of measurement Ordered categories are not coded in the same direction (e.g. as needed to produce a composite scale or index), or the codes do not match the quantity their categories imply (e.g. higher codes for higher income groups)	• Reorder the categories (e.g. by frequency, similarity, or rank order) • Recode the categories; e.g. reverse code them so that they are all coded in the same required direction
It is unclear whether non-committal responses (e.g. 'don't know') indicate ambivalence or non-attitudes, making these responses difficult to manage	• Reconceptualize the variable (e.g. from 'yes', 'no', 'don't know', to 'yes' and 'other')
Outliers (atypical numeric values in a variable's distribution) distort the results	• Transform the variable (through mathematical functions) or delete the variable

Table 6.11 (Continued)

Problem	Remedy at the data analysis stage
A selection bias is detected that distorts the results	Adjust for the bias: • Use statistical methods (partial correlations or multivariate analysis) to remove the effect of the bias variable on a relationship between variables • Calculate and apply weights, for example:

	Sample	Population
Male	30%	45%
Female	70%	55%

Problem	Remedy at the data analysis stage
	Weight = Population % / Sample %; thus the weight for males is 45/30 = 1.5, and the weight for females is 55/70 = 0.79. Apply the weight in our data analysis • Manage bias due to 'missing values' by dropping cases or imputing a value to replace the missing values
Continuous variables are not related in a straight line	• Take no action if we are presenting our findings as crosstabulations or as a table of means • Summarize the relationship using a correlation coefficient sensitive to the non-linearity • Transform the curve summarizing the relationship
Continuous variables deviate greatly from a 'normal distribution' (bell-shaped curve)	• Use an equivalent non-parametric statistic (Table 6.12) • Transform the variable to make it normal and permit the use of parametric statistics; e.g. cube the variable to adjust for a severe negative skew (long left hand tail)
Which test to use is unclear	• See Table 6.13
Confounding bias is detected	• Adjust for the bias through standardization, stratified analysis or statistical modeling

Sometimes, we can make processing errors by using parametric instead of non-parametric methods of analysis. Parametric (or classical) methods (or tests) analyze interval level (continuous) sample data that are assumed to come from a background population with a recognizable probability distribution (most typically one that is approximately normal). However, when this assumption cannot be reasonably made – especially when the samples tested are small – we need to consider using non-parametric (distribution-free) methods. These methods are less powerful than parametric methods but can be applied to nominal, ordinal or interval level data. Table 6.12 lists parametric tests, and non-parametric alternatives, for different research purposes. Table 6.13 suggests how to use the measurement level of two variables to select appropriate descriptive statistical tests [11].

Table 6.12. Parametric (normal distribution) and non-Parametric (non-normal Distribution) Statistical Tests for Describing Continuous Variables

Purpose of test	Example	Parametric test (look at absolute differences between values)	Non-parametric alternative (these look at the rank order of values)
Compare differences between 2 independent groups	Compare boys' ages with girls' ages	t test (two-sample, unpaired)	Mann-Whitney U test
Compare differences between 3+ independent groups	Compare the Body Mass Indexes of Catholics, Protestants and Jews	One-way analysis of variance	Kruskall-Wallis analysis of ranks
Assess the strength and direction of the linear relationship between 2 variables	Assess the relationship between platelet count and C-reactive protein	Pearson's correlation coefficient	Spearman's rank order correlation coefficient; also, e.g., Kendall's tau, Gamma
Compare differences between 2 measures on a single sample group	Compare number of visits to a doctor before and after treatment	t test (one-sample, paired)	Wilcoxon matched pairs test
Compare 3+ measures on a single sample group	Compare plasma glucose levels 1, 2 and 3 hours after easting	One way analysis of variance	Kruskall-Wallis analysis of variance by ranks
As above, but test the influence (and interaction) of two different covariates	As above, but look at whether results differ between males and females	Two-way analysis of variance	Two-way analysis of variance by ranks

Table 6.13. Selecting Appropriate Descriptive Statistical Procedures

Measurement level of first variable	Single variable procedure	Two-variable (bivariate) procedure Measurement level of second variable			
		Dichotomy	Nominal	Ordinal	Interval (and ratio)
Dichotomy	Proportions, percentages, ratios	Difference of proportions, Phi, Chi-square, Fishers exact test,			
Nominal	Proportions, percentages, mode, ratios	Cramér's V, Lamda, Chi-square	Cramer's V, Lamda, Goodman and Kruskall's tau, Chi-square		
Ordinal	Medians, quartiles, deciles, interquartile range	Mann-Whitney, runs, Smirnov, signed ranks, Rank-biserial	Friedman's analysis of variance with ranks	Kendall's tau, Gamma, Rank-order	
Interval (and ratio)	Means, medians, variance, standard deviations	Difference of means, Point-biserial	Analysis of variance	Spearman's r, multiserial correlation	Pearson's correlation, and regression

REFERENCES

[1]   McColl E, A Jacoby A, Thomas L, Soutter J, Bamford C, Steen N, et al. Design and use of questionnaires: a review of best practice applicable to surveys of health service staff and patients. *Health Technology Assessment* 2001;5(31).

[2]   Bradburn N, Sudman S, Wansink B. *Asking questions: the definitive guide to questionnaire design for market research, political polls, and social and health questionnaires.* San Francisco Jossey-Bass, 2004.

[3]   Kendall K, Kendall J. *Systems analysis and design.* 4th Edition. Englewood Cliffs, NJ: Prentice Hall, 1998.

[4]   Bowling A. Techniques of questionnaire design. In: Bowling A, Ebrahim S, editors. *Handbook of Health Research Methods.* Maidenhead: Open University Press, 2005:394-427.

[5]   Fowler F, Mangione T. *Standardized Survey Interviewing. Minimizing Interviewer-Related Error.* Thousand Oaks, CA: Sage, 1990.

[6]   Weisberg H. *The Total Survey Error Approach.* Chicago: University of Chicago Press, 2005.

[7]   Carr M. Who cares about empathy? *Second opinion* 2001;7:73-82.

[8]   McCracken G. *The Long Interview.* Newbury Park, CA: Sage, 1988.

[9]   De Vaus D. *Analyzing Social Science Data.* London: Sage Publications, 2002.

[10]   Good P, Hardin J. *Common Errors in Statistics (and How to Avoid Them).* Hoboken, NJ: John Wiley and Sons, Inc, 2003.

[11]   Blalock H. *Social Statistics.* 2nd Edition. Tokyo: McGraw HIll, 1979.

Chapter 7

RANDOMIZED CONTROLLED TRIALS

OBJECTIVES

By the time you have completed this chapter, you should be able to:

1. Define the concept of randomized controlled trials
2. Discuss ethical considerations relevant to randomized trials
3. Report limitations of randomized trials
4. Describe types of clinical trials
5. Evaluate different design classifications of randomized trials
6. Access electronic support for estimating sample sizes for these trials
7. List what to include in reporting the trials
8. Critically appraise a randomized trial paper

PREVIEW

Because of its ability to minimize random error and bias, the randomized controlled trial (or more simply, the randomized trial) is usually considered to be the gold standard for evaluating health care interventions, particularly in terms of their relative effectiveness. In Chapter 2, the discussion on 'choosing study designs' indicated that this belief may too simplistic, not because we overvalue randomized trials but because we undervalue well-conducted observational studies. Chapter 2 also introduced PECOT as a framework for developing focused questions that we can answer using designs such as randomized trials. This current Chapter builds on that discussion by providing the basic knowledge and skills needed to review critically, design carefully and conduct properly a randomized trial. It also elaborates on limitations of this design and notes issues relevant to applying trial findings.

DESCRIPTION AND PURPOSE OF RANDOMIZED CONTROLLED TRIALS

A randomized trial is an experiment (Figure 2.1 and Table 2.2) that aims to answer a primary question relating usually to the relative effectiveness (or efficacy) of an intervention. In a randomized trial the investigators artificially control the conditions for measurement. They construct two or more groups, including an (experimental) intervention group and a control (intervention) group. The main types of control groups are placebo concurrent control and active treatment concurrent control. Randomization is the preferred method of allocation to the intervention groups. It controls for selection bias; tends to balance the groups on known and unknown characteristics, making the groups likely to differ only on the intervention allocated; and guarantees the validity of classical tests of statistical significance. Relevant outcomes (and group characteristics) are measured at the start of the study. After sufficient follow-up, outcomes are compared with each other to estimate the relative effectiveness of the interventions. Any outcome difference between the groups is attributed to the intervention (the effect).

There has to be genuine uncertainty about, and a need to know, the postulated effect of the intervention in order to justify a randomized trial. Moreover, the study question and any secondary or subsidiary questions should be important; carefully and clearly formulated; feasible to answer; and stated in advance (see Chapter 2) for a study population also specified in advance. Randomized trials are most appropriate when the effect size of the intervention is expected to be only modest.

CONSTRAINTS ON CONDUCTING A TRIAL

In Chapter 2, we looked at factors challenging the use of evidence hierarchies, which, as noted above, locate randomized trials at the apex for study designs to evaluate interventions. We will now elaborate on constraints to conducting randomized trials. Some of these constraints are pragmatic. For example, randomized trials can be expensive to conduct and be unwieldy as illustrated by challenges in recruiting and retaining centers and participants. Meeting such challenges requires careful planning, using the simplest design possible, and adequately resourcing trials to answer important questions [1].

Concerns about the ethics of randomized trials are also pervasive. Among the most important ethical (and scientific) requirements for starting randomized trials is collective uncertainty (equipoise), among health experts, about the preferred intervention. Other ethical concerns may relate to the potential to violate participants' rights. However, such concerns typically result from poor trial design and conduct in specific circumstances. Table 7.1 notes key ethical concerns and how to manage them.

Table 7.2 elaborates on barriers to conducting randomized trials. It summarizes when randomized trials may be unnecessary, inappropriate, impossible or inadequate [3]. In these circumstances, well-controlled observational studies offer one solution; the table suggests others.

Table 7.1. Ethics of Randomized Trials

Issue	Concern	Response
Role of well-conducted observational studies in the evaluation of interventions	Overestimation of the ability of randomized trials to contribute to knowledge about effectiveness [2]. Downgrading of well-conducted observational studies for the purpose of evaluation	See Table 7.2
Experimenters act to acquire generalizable scientific knowledge for the collective good rather than exclusively for any individual participant	Participants need to understand that the likelihood of personal benefit is low	Obtain participants' informed consent (even though the same standard is not set for interventions of uncertain benefit in routine clinical practice). Practice based on unproven interventions is unethical
Trials may expose participants to risks of harm	Participants may not be fully informed of, or understand, the risks of participating in the trial	Obtain participants' informed consent. The extent to which vulnerable participants can give this consent is moot. But this problem is not unique to trials
Randomization allocates participants according to chance alone	Professionals ought to have a preference for each participant's intervention, even when the research evidence favors no particular intervention	'Equipoise' (genuine uncertainty) and the need to remove bias justify randomization. Monitor changes in equipoise to stop trials when necessary
Participants may have firm preferences for a particular intervention	Allocation to another intervention group may weaken adherence, promote withdrawal from the study, and lead to strong dissatisfaction	Participants with firm preferences are not eligible to take part in these trials; an exception is preference trials (see Table 7.6)
Some trials require placebo controls	Placebo controls are unethical when an effective intervention exists	Evaluate the experimental intervention against the available, standard (usual) intervention

Table 7.2. Limitations of Randomized Trials

Situation	Reason	Example	Solutions other than observational studies
Experimentation may be 'unnecessary'	• Intervention produces such a large effect that the effect of unknown confounding can be ignored	• Penicillin for bacterial infections; insulin in type 1 diabetes	• Safety trials
	• 'Successful interventions for otherwise fatal conditions' and when it is not feasible to wait to conduct a randomized trial [4]	• Vaccination against an epidemic of Meningococcal B disease, for example in New Zealand	
	• Well-conducted observational studies compared with randomized trials might not systematically overestimate the size of intervention effects on the same topic [5 6]	• Screening for breast cancer. Despite critics [7], some pro-mammography public policies are strongly influenced by the observational evidence [8]	
Experimentation may be 'inappropriate'	• Intervention is rapidly changing	• Historically, anti-retroviral treatments for HIV	• 'Small' randomized trials following a Bayesian approach [10]
	• Infrequent adverse outcomes	• Rare adverse drug effects	• Mega-trials involving several thousand participants
	• Interventions to treat rare events	• Treatment of rare cancers	
	• Interventions to prevent rare events are difficult to evaluate	• Lying infants supine or on their side to prevent Sudden Infant Death Syndrome	
	• Outcomes are far in the future	• Long term consequences of oral contraceptives	• Long-term follow-up
	• Random allocation may reduce effectiveness that depends on subjects' active participation [3]	• Clinical audit	• Preference arms
	• Small differences in the intervention effects (and sometimes high costs)	• Use of a statin for primary prevention in low-risk patients [9]	

Table 7.2 (Continued)

Situation	Reason	Example	Solutions other than observational studies
Experimentation may be 'impossible'	• Clinicians and others may refuse to take part, e.g. if they believe that their own practice style is correct	• Trial of effectiveness of surgery for stress incontinence	• Persuasion • Address collective *and* individual equipoise • Develop acceptable methods of allocation • Keep consent procedures and data collection as simple as possible
	• Ethical objections • Political obstacles • Legal obstacles	• Intensive care v. ward care • GP fundholding in the UK • Private sector ophthalmologists blocked a trial of radial keratotomy • Referrals to more distant facilities	• Persuasion • Persuasion
	• Some interventions cannot be allocated randomly		
	• Contamination	• Clinicians being expected to provide care in more than one way	• Cluster randomization. Expertise trials that randomize subjects to clinicians with expertise in either intervention A or intervention B [11]
	• So many interventions in use that it will be never be possible to subject them all to experimental evaluation		• Increasing the funding available for experiments will be of some help
Experimentation may be 'inadequate'	• Lack of generalizability to local settings. Also, lack of applicability to individual participants or groups who differ from the group average	• Anticoagulation treatment for atrial fibrillation [12]. The potential for benefit or, in this example, for harm (major hemorrhage) may depend on attributes of the participants, setting or intervention. Variation in these produces heterogeneity of intervention effects	• Undertake pragmatic trials. Apply the fixed benefit in trial(s) to the baseline risk • Withhold final approval of marketed treatments until there is evidence of their effects in population subgroups [13] • Answer, in context, questions on biologic, social and economic, and epidemiologic issues guide clinical decisions on when trial results apply to individual participants [14]
	• May lack internal validity	• Differential expertise bias (for example, clinicians have more expertise in treatment A than treatment B)	• Expertise based trials [11]

STAGES OF A CLINICAL TRIAL

Some randomized trials are clinical trials. Before these randomized trials can be undertaken as formal comparative studies, the clinical trials may need to progress through other stages of development. Table 7.3 categorizes different trials in the context of these design stages.

It is important to register clinical trials before enrolling the first patient. This is required by members of the International Committee of Medical Journal Editors to produce a comprehensive, publicly available database of clinical trials that can be considered for publication [15].

Table 7.3. Clinical Trial Design by Development Stage

Stage of development	Purpose	Characteristic	Equivalent phase in therapeutic drug development
Early development studies	Test an intervention mechanism, for example the bioavailability of a drug. Undertake dose-finding	Close connection to biologic models	Phase I trial
Middle development studies	Determine feasibility, and assess safety and efficacy	Pivotal to intervention development	Phase II trial
Comparative studies	Assess comparative intervention efficacy	Use concurrent controls. Pivotal to intervention regulation	Phase III trial
Late development studies	Undertake an expanded safety assessment, for example of uncommon effects of the intervention	Large-scale	Phase IV trial (or post-marketing surveillance studies)

DESIGN CLASSIFICATIONS

The design of randomized trials can be classified in numerous ways. Tables 7.4-7.14 display eight different design classifications.

Philosophy

Different philosophies underlie what it is considered most important for randomized trials to find out, and how. Typically, depending on whether the orientation of the investigators is on effectiveness as an ideal or as a practical application, randomized trials may be labeled either pragmatic trials or explanatory trials (Table 7.4) [16]. In practice, however, most randomized trials contain elements of each of these types; thus the challenge is less usually to select one, rather than the other, than to select the best combination of their elements to answer the study question.

Table 7.4. Randomized Trial Designs According to Philosophy

Type	Pragmatic trials (also called management trials)	Explanatory trials
Description	Focus on 'use-effectiveness' to inform choices between treatments Show (a) whether the intervention works under 'real-life' conditions (is effective), from a participant perspective, and (b) consequences of its use	• Focus on 'method- effectiveness' to further scientific knowledge Demonstrate whether an intervention 'works' under ideal or selected conditions (is efficacious) and, if so, how and why
Intervention	Apply wide inclusion criteria. May permit variations in treatment; i.e. loose control (e.g. flexible dosing regimen), and be at the discretion of the routine clinical staff	• Are strictly defined (e.g. fixed dosing regimens) and controlled by the investigators • Need highly trained staff
Control	Select active control (e.g. new anti-hypertensive v. beta-blocker) as usually used in routine practice; placebos are seldom used	• Often use placebos
Participant selection criteria	Select heterogeneous groups of participants to reflect routine practice	• Apply strict eligibility criteria to produce highly homogenous groups
Blinding	May or may not permit blinding	• Usually involve blinding
Outcome	Represent the full range of health gains. Can include 'hard' outcomes as well as 'soft' outcomes such as quality of life	• Focus on 'hard' outcomes, such as blood pressure. • Often use intermediate outcomes
Analysis	Usually analyze by intention to treat	• Analyze by intention to treat
(Dis)advantages	Can show what services to provide, but tend to give limited insights into how or why the intervention works or not	• Can reveal how or why an intervention works. • Cannot indicate whether to provide it to a wide range of participants in different settings

Unit of Randomization

Tables 7.5-7.14 summarize other ways of classifying the designs of randomized trials. The tables show how these designs vary according to a range of methodological criteria, including the unit of randomization (Table 7.5) and method of allocating participants to intervention groups (Table 7.6), including the permuted (or randomized) block method (Table 7.7) and minimization (Table 7.8). Careful consideration of all these criteria is important because how randomized trials are designed will influence, usually from the outset, their ability to satisfy ethical constraints, reduce error and control precision.

Table 7.5. Randomized Trial Designs According to the Unit of Randomization

Design	Description	Rationale	Advantages	Disadvantages
Conventional individual randomization	Randomizes the *individual* participants, for example either to Intervention A or to Intervention B	No risk of contamination across trial groups	• Straightforward to design and analyze; efficient	• Inefficient when the risk of contamination > 30%. Increase the sample size to manage this problem
(1) Expertise-based trial	Randomizes individual participants to clinicians with expertise in intervention A or intervention B respectively	Potential for 'differential expertise bias' in providing intervention A or B	• May enhance the validity feasibility and ethics of randomized trials of non-pharmacological interventions, such as physiotherapy	• Experts might not be available to take part within the same trial sites
Cluster (or group) randomization	Randomizes *groups* of participants (such as practices) to the different study interventions	Risk of contamination across trial groups (e.g. in a trial of dietary change, control participants could learn about and adopt the experimental diet)	• Minimizes within the same cluster the risk of control participants being exposed to, and adopting, the experimental intervention	• Potential for recruitment bias • More complex to design and analyze • Requires more participants to retain statistical power

Table 7.6. Randomized Trial Designs According to How Participants Are Allocated to Intervention Groups

Design	Description	Example	Rationale	Advantages	Disadvantages
Fixed allocation					
A. Complete (simple) randomized design	Randomizes participants, without restriction, to the study interventions; i.e. their allocation is independent of all previous allocations	Each participant is randomized to either simvastatin (group A) or placebo (group B)	Can avoid selection bias and control for all confounding factors in a probabilistic sense	• Minimizes bias in the allocation of participants • Is flexible and easy to implement	• Risks a large imbalance occurring in the number or characteristics of participants randomized to each intervention group
B. Restricted (to balance the groups in size or characteristics)	Randomizes participants, to meet a required ratio (e.g. 1:1), in an intervention block of specified size	See Table 7.7 below	Helps to maintain balance in the numbers allocated to each intervention group during the trial	• Aids comparability • Protects against unequal numbers if the trial is small or is terminated before participant enrolment is completed	• Reduces the unpredictability of the allocation sequence if known, small block sizes are used. Therefore, it is best to vary the block size during recruitment
1. Block (permuted block) design	Free software at:www.cancerbiostats.onc.jhmi.edu/software.cfm generates randomized treatment assignments that are blocked, and optionally stratified				
2. Stratification	Separately randomizes participants (usually with blocking) within each of two or more strata of participants		As above but within each stratum separately of the confounding variable	• Can hold confounding factors constant	• Increases the comparability of the study groups, especially in small trials

Table 7.6 (Continued)

Design	Description	Example	Rationale	Advantages	Disadvantages
Adaptive (dynamic) randomization designs					
A. Restricted	Checks the previous allocation of similar participants. Makes the next allocation to best balance the intervention groups, across all the stratification variables	See below	Adapts the allocation probabilities to imbalances caused by randomization.	• Responds to data collected during the trial • Maximizes the impact of each participant's contribution to the trial	• See below
1. Baseline adaptive randomization	Adapts allocation probabilities to imbalances in the numbers of participants, or in baseline characteristics	(a) Urn design	Improves balance		• Produces a loss of power
		(b) Minimization	Yields tight balance		• Key, immediately occurring response variable may not exist • Complicates analysis
(a) Minimization	Allocates the first participant randomly. Assigns each subsequent participant to the group minimizing the imbalance between the groups on specified prognostic factors	See Table 7.8 below	Achieves balance between intervention groups for specified prognostic factors	• Can produce more balance than do blocked strata • Yields unbiased estimates of the treatment effect	• Requires the researcher to keep track of the current measure of imbalance
2. Response adaptive randomization	Adapts allocation probabilities to imbalances on participants' responses to the intervention group	Play the winner	Maximizes the number of participants receiving the 'superior' intervention		• Can be very difficult to carry out and analyze

Table 7.6 (Continued)

Design	Description	Example	Rationale	Advantages	Disadvantages
Preference designs					
1. Comprehensive cohort (Brewin–Bradley) design	Lets participants decide to be randomized or else choose their intervention group	Each participant either chooses to be randomized to counseling (group A) or no counseling (group B), or chooses to receive counseling (group C) or no counseling (group D)	Accommodates strong intervention preferences that can otherwise lead to a refusal to be randomized or, in the absence of blinding, to poor adherence to an allocated but unwanted intervention	• Can show both the effect of the study interventions, and the additional influence of motivational factors.	• Exposes the preference groups to selection bias. It is unclear how to compare the findings involving the preference groups
2. Zelen's (single randomized consent) design	Randomizes participants before they give consent. Only those randomized to the experimental intervention are informed and invited to give consent. If they decline, they receive the control intervention but are analyzed as if getting the experimental group		Aids recruitment	• Increases participation • Tends to increase compliance; resembles actual clinical practice	• Introduces ethical concerns • Lacks blinding • Reduces the study power if a large proportion decline the experimental intervention offered
3. Double randomized consent	Tells all participants the group to which they have been randomized. They can then switch		Addresses the problem of not seeking informed consent from the control group, and be suitable when there is no best standard (control) intervention	• Helps to fulfill the requirements of the rationale	• Can weaken the statistical power of the trial • Does not permit double blinding • Leaves the consenting process still unclear
4. Wennberg's (two-arm trial) design [18]	Randomizes eligible participants to a 'randomized controlled trial group' or a preference (free choice) group		Estimates the impact of participant preferences on the outcomes	• Can reveal from, between-group comparisons, how preferences influence the study outcome	• Is complex, requires large numbers and is time-consuming • The preference group may not have strong preferences; the randomized group may have strong preferences

Table 7.7. Permuted Block Method of Randomization
(For A Block Size of 4, Where A = Experimental Intervention and B = Control Intervention [17])

Random number sequence	Permuted blocks	Randomization list	
1	1. AABB	1	A A B B
3	2. ABAB		
9	3. ABBA	3	A B B A
5	4. BBAA		
8	5. BABA	5	B A B A
(Etc)	6. BAAB		

Table 7.8. Example of randomization using the minimization method (In a trial of two health assessment methods among community-dwelling older people, with stratification factors of age, gender and area of residence)

Characteristic	Intervention A	Intervention B
70-84	8	10
85+	10	8
Female	5	7
Male	13	11
Urban	9	10
Rural	9	8
Total	18	18

The next participant (no. 37) has the following characteristics: 85+, female, rural area. Subtotals for the intervention allocation to this attribute profile are $10 + 5 + 9 = 24$ for Intervention A and $8 + 7 + 8 = 23$ for Intervention B (note that participants are counted more than once). Participant no. 37 would therefore be allocated to Intervention B. When the tallies on A and B are equal within a profile, randomly allocate the next participant. This process is equivalent to a permuted block size of two within the profile

Allocation Scheme

Intervention allocation schemes aim to reduce bias, produce balanced comparisons and estimate error. Three main types of schemes are used. (1) In *fixed allocations schemes*, assignments to the intervention groups are made with a pre-specified (usually equal) probability. The allocations may involve either simple randomization or, to balance the intervention groups, constrained (restricted) randomization; the constraints include blocking and stratification. (2) By adjusting allocation probabilities as a trial progresses, *adaptive (dynamic) randomization schemes* also restrict randomization. (3) *Preference designs* can incorporate the intervention preferences of eligible, non-randomized participants. However, an alternative is to elicit preferences before randomization, randomize all participants regardless of their preferences, and include preferences in the analysis.

Exposure Type

Randomized trial designs can be distinguished by variation in the type of exposure by participants to the study interventions. Table 7.9 summarizes four of the most important designs, the most common of which is the parallel trial.

PARTICIPANT NUMBERS

As Table 7.10 shows, randomized trials can be designed to vary in size, from individual participant (n of 1) trials to large, simple trials (mega-trials). Trial sizes may or may not be fixed at the outset.

Table 7.9. Randomized Trial Designs According to the Type of Exposure to the Study Interventions

Design	Description	Example	Rationale	Advantages	Disadvantages
Parallel (group) design	Allocates each participant independently to only one study intervention	Each participant receives either intervention A or intervention B	Permits a *between* participants-comparison of the effect an experimental intervention versus a control intervention	• Is straightforward, makes few assumptions, and permits valid comparisons	• Is inefficient, for example in size, time and cost
Withdrawal trial	Randomizes each participant, who has been treated for a fixed period, to continue the test treatment (or different dosages) or to placebo.	Assesses responses to discontinuation or reduction of treatment.	• Can rule out placebo effects • Shows the duration of benefit of the active treatment	• Requires care with withdrawal • Risks selection bias • Participants and disease states can change	
Cross-over design	Randomizes each participant (in a random sequence) to each study intervention in successive periods	After receiving intervention A in period 1, the participant 'crosses over' to receive intervention B in period 2, or vice versa	Permits comparisons *within* participants. Since participants act as their own controls, valid results require fewer participants	• Can efficiently assess rapid effects of short duration on chronic, stable and permanently alterable conditions	• Can, without a washout period, 'carry over' effects of one intervention,' changing the effect of subsequent interventions • Prone to 'period' effects (time or season observed)
Factorial design	Compares two or more experimental interventions separately, in combination, and against a control	Participants receive intervention A + placebo B; intervention B + placebo A; intervention A + intervention B; or placebo A + placebo B	Permits comparisons of the independent and interaction effects of two experimental interventions in a single trial	• Can efficiently address two or more questions at the same time	• Is complex • Generally has low power to detect interactions

Table 7.10. Randomized Trial Designs According to the Number of Participants

Design	Description	Rationale	Advantages	Disadvantages
n-of-1 (individual participant) trial	Is a form of cross-over trial. One participant receives separately and in random order the experimental and control interventions on two or more occasions	Determines the most effective intervention in an individual case.	• Is useful when multi-participant clinical trials are unavailable, or do not apply to a particular case, and blinding is possible	• Is limited to participants with chronic, stable conditions. Intervention effects should be rapid and reverse on stopping the intervention • Carry-over and period effects can occur
Large, simple trial (mega-trial)	Is a pragmatic trial that collects limited data from thousands of participants across many trial sites	Provides reliable evidence of moderate, clinically important effects of relatively easily administered interventions	• Makes it unnecessary to select participants carefully at entry • Produces precise and generalizable results	• Must be kept simple to be feasible • Cannot easily manage complex outcomes • Usually requires a relatively short period of follow-up
Fixed size trial	Fixes the sample size at the outset. The intention is to enroll and follow this number of participants	Ensures at the outset that the trial has adequate statistical power.	• Can avoid problems in managing and interpreting sequential trial data	• Need a good measure of the variance in the outcome of key interest • May lack flexibility, involve delays and tie up resources
Sequential trial design	Does not specify the number of participants before the trial begins. Analyzes data as they become available, until a positive, negative, or no effect becomes clear	Stops the trial as soon as the effects of the interventions become clear	• Compared with fixed size trials, is shorter, on average, with fewer participants; 'closed sequential designs' put an upper bound on enrolment	• Is limited to conditions where a single outcome of primary interest is known soon after the trial begins • Multiple comparisons may require a larger sample than for a fixed size trial

Table 7.11. Randomized Trial Designs According to the Level of Blinding

Design	Description	Advantages	Disadvantages
Unblinded (open) trial	Blinds no-one. All participants and investigators know who has been allocated to which treatment group	• Can be easier to do than blinded trials • Helps investigators to make decisions, e.g. on whether to continue individual participants on their intervention	• Has the potential for bias, particularly when the outcome is subjective, and for a high dropout rate among the participants not receiving the experimental intervention
Single-blind trial	Blinds only one party to the treatment allocation	• As above • Partially reduces bias • May best protect participants' health	• As above, though less pronounced
Double-blind trial	Blinds participants and investigators to the treatment allocation	• Can minimize bias • May be more ethical than the trials with less blinding	• Is more complex and costly than open or single-blind designs (e.g. may require emergency unblinding procedures or using the 'double dummy' method to compare different active interventions) • Is usually feasible only for drug trials • May never fully remove bias
Triple or quadruple-blind design	Blinds participants and investigators plus the data management staff/committee monitoring the study outcomes do not know participants' group allocation	• Helps the monitoring committee to assess the results objectively	• Does not usually allow the monitoring committee to make informed decisions, on time, about individual participants [19]

Table 7.12. Randomized Trial Designs According to Trial Endpoints

Type of endpoint	Description	Example	Advantages	Disadvantages
'Hard' endpoint	Objective and quantifiable	Death	• May offer accurate and repeatable measurement	• May not be relevant to preferred endpoints
'Soft' endpoint	Subjective	Self-reported functional status	• High clinical relevance	• Subjective and may have low reliability
True endpoint (clinical outcome)	Clinically most meaningful endpoint	Myocardial infarction (MI) or death from MI	• Direct measure of clinical benefit	• May be inaccessible owing to time, cost or difficulty of measurement
Surrogate endpoint	Substitutes for, and predicts, the true endpoint	Serum cholesterol level	• Accessible. Reduces completion time, sample size, and cost	• Must be validated as causally connected to, and capturing all effects of the interventions on, the true endpoint
Individual endpoint	Single clinical outcome	All-cause mortality	• Insufficient statistical power to estimate an intervention's true effect	• Easily interpretable
Composite endpoint	Cluster of clinically related outcomes	All-cause mortality: death from cardiovascular event; myocardial infarction and stroke	• Overcomes the problem of insufficient power (e.g. to study rare diseases or complete the trial in a feasible timeframe)	• Can yield conflicting results • Depends, for its valid interpretation, on the similarity in: the importance of each component outcome; the effects of the interventions; and the number of events across components [20]
Endpoint defined by data characteristics	Continuous endpoints Event times Counts Dichotomies Other categorical endpoints	Serum cholesterol level Time to hospital discharge Number of clinic visits in one year Survival or death Cancer staging	• It is best to select a rigorously defined endpoint whose measurement, with established reliability and validity, is most relevant to the participants and to answering the research question most efficiently using the data available	
Special endpoints	Health-related quality of life	See Table 7.13	• Can validly and reliably measure participant experiences and perceptions of life quality in relation to the interventions	• Subjective and prone to measurement error.

Table 7.13. Measures of Patients' Health-Related Quality of Life (HRQL)

These are standardized, patient-assessed measures of one or more dimensions of the quality of life influenced by ill-health or treatment

Alternative names	Applications	Types	Examples	Advantages	Disadvantages
Health status measures	Outcome in evaluative research	Generic	Short-Form-36 (SF-36)	• Reflect the patient perspective	• HRQL can have different meanings, on which precise agreement is lacking
Subjective health status indicators	Health needs assessments	Disease-specific	Seattle Angina Questionnaire	• Patient assessed measures may disagree with proxy measures produced by service providers	• Variation in the aims, concepts, domains, formats and analysis of these measures
Functional status measures	Resource allocation	Dimension-specific	Arthritis Impact Measurement Scale		• Same disadvantages as can weaken other health measures, such as low validity
Patient-assessed outcome measures	Audit and quality assurance	Population-specific	PedsQL		• Subjective measures reduce precision and tend to reflect researcher priorities
Quality of life measures	Clinical care of individual patients	Site or region-specific	Roland-Morris Questionnaire on Back Pain		• HRQL measures may not be sensitive to minor disorders or the small impact of an intervention

Blinding

Blinding is different from *allocation concealment*. Concealment of the intervention allocation for each participant (ideally through a centralized or remote service for randomization) protects the assignment sequence *before and until allocation*. It shields people in a trial from knowing future assignments in advance. It thereby helps to remove selection bias associated with who gets into the trial and which intervention they get.

In contrast, blinding (also called masking) seeks, *after the intervention allocation,* to conceal the assignment from the investigators and participants. This aims to prevent systematic modification of their behavior (ascertainment bias), e.g. a change in participant response to the intervention and reporting of its effect, or in clinician management of a participant. Table 7.11 assesses different levels of blinding of randomized trials.

Endpoints

Randomized trials should have a primary endpoint (primary outcome). Table 7.12 evaluates the different types of endpoint. This quantitative measure is the most meaningful, planned outcomes of the trial intervention for participants. It should be described in, and used to meet, the trial objectives. However, changing the primary endpoint during the study may be appropriate if doing so is based on the overall event rate in the whole study cohort and not on knowing interim results of the effect of the study interventions. Secondary endpoints can contribute to the interpretation of trial findings. Endpoints must be relevant and properly measured. Table 7.13 focuses on measures of one endpoint: health-related quality of life (HRQL). It may be noted that health state utilities assess through health indices the value that people place on particular health states but are not, in themselves, measures of HRQL.

Method of Analysis

The research question should guide the trial strategy and method of analysis. Faced with data imperfections resulting from protocol non-adherence, investigators most commonly choose to analyze their trial data according to 'intention-to-treat.' Alternative approaches to analysis, whose value should probably be determined on a study-by-study basis, include 'treatment-received' (Table 7.14). However, it is possible to reconcile these approaches by carefully defining the eligibility criteria and only entering participants into the trial if they can be reasonably expected to complete the allocated intervention.

Study interventions should be compared at the end of the study for effectiveness shown through 'differences (e.g. between means or medians, proportions), ratios of quantities measuring association (odds, risk, hazards) or ratios of quantities measuring effect (variances or correlations).' [21] To this end, readers need sufficient information to calculate endpoints in different formats. For example, reporting the number of participants that experienced the event of interest in each group and the number at risk in each group allows readers to calculate and compare the proportion in each group experiencing the event (risk) and, in turn, the difference in proportions (absolute risk difference). Dividing the risk difference by the risk in the control group yields the commonly reported effect measure: the relative risk reduction (see Table 2.8). Confidence intervals and p values can also be readily calculated. [21]

In addition, interim data analyses may be needed for treatment (safety) monitoring (of unexpected adverse effects) over the life of the trial. The monitoring (which should accompany checking for protocol compliance) should be the same in all study groups and not outweigh the intervention processes. It may also indicate data deficiencies and inform the selection of the method of data analysis.

Table 7.14. Randomized Trial Designs According to the Method of Analysis

	Intention-to-treat	Treatment (intervention) received [22]
Description	Analyzes all participants according to the intervention group to which they were allocated, regardless of which intervention they received or their continuation in the trial	Analyzes participants according to the intervention they received, regardless of the intervention they were originally allocated
Perspective	Tests treatment policy. It assesses effects of recommending or offering an intervention and starting participants on it	Tests the intervention received; i.e. tests what happens when participants adhere to the intervention they were allocated
Approach	Experimental and pragmatic	Explanatory
Rationale	Meets the statistical need for unbiased estimation and correct error levels	Meets the clinical need to estimate effects of the interventions
Strength	Permits a valid test of the null hypothesis of no intervention difference. Reflects the clinical reality of treatment non-adherence and protocol deviations	May accurately estimate the effect of the allocated interventions, and can adjust for known causes of crossover
Limitations	Estimates the intervention effects conservatively, and can be difficult to interpret if significant crossover occurs. Is not fully applicable when outcome data are missing for some participants	Compromises the effect of random allocation by excluding non-adherent participants. Differential dropout rates between groups can also produce misleading results. May not represent the practical impact of the intervention plan
Reporting	Describes handling of deviations from random allocation and of missing data on the primary outcome variable	Clearly states assumptions made and the potential for bias

SAMPLE SIZE ESTIMATION

Early in designing a randomized trial, we usually need to estimate the sample size (number of experimental subjects) needed to answer our primary question (although see Table 7.10). The sample must be large enough to have the statistical power to detect differences in our primary endpoint, between the intervention groups, which are substantively (e.g. clinically) and statistically significant. At the same time, the sample size estimated must be feasible to obtain and not too large (which would expose many participants to the less effective intervention and waste research time, participant effort and support costs).

Various texts [19] describe the statistical calculations involved in estimating sample sizes. However, computer programs simplify the calculations. For example, software at: www.cancerbiostats.onc.jhmi.edu/software.cfm is freely available to calculate the statistical power and sample size needed for clinical trials. Perhaps easier to use is the calculator at: http://hedwig.mgh.harvard.edu/sample_size/size.html which estimates the sample size, statistical power, or minimum detectable difference for three types of response variable (dichotomous, continuous, or time to event) according to three trial designs (parallel design, crossover design, and trials to find associations between variables). It also produces a paragraph from the output. Since assumptions underpinning the calculations do not hold for all trials, the developers recommend consulting a biostatistician when planning a trial.

REPORTING

The CONSORT (Consolidated Standards of Reporting Trials) statement [23] (Table 7.15) and its extension to cluster trials [24] are initiatives to improve the reporting and interpretation of the design, methods and results of randomized trials. A recent systematic review [25] concluded that journal endorsement of the CONSORT statement for parallel-group randomized trials is associated with improved reporting of these trials. The CONSORT guidelines help us to structure reporting of randomized trials and critical appraisal of the trials reported by others.

Table 7.15. Consort Checklist of Items to Include When Reporting a Randomized Trial [23]

Topic	Description
TITLE and ABSTRACT	How participants were allocated to interventions (*e.g.*, "random allocation", "randomized", or "randomly assigned")
INTRODUCTION Background	Scientific background and explanation of rationale
METHODS Participants	Eligibility criteria for participants and the settings and locations where the data were collected
Interventions	Precise details of the intervention intended for each group and how and when they were actually determined
Objectives	Specific objectives and hypotheses
Outcomes	Clearly defined primary and secondary outcome measures and, when applicable, any methods used to enhance the quality of measurements (*e.g.*, multiple observations, training of assessors)
Sample size	How sample size was determined and, when applicable, explanation of any interim analyses and stopping rules
Randomization -- Sequence generation	Method used to generate the random allocation sequence, including details of any restrictions (*e.g.*, blocking, stratification)
Randomization -- Allocation concealment	Method used to implement the random allocation sequence (*e.g.*, numbered containers or central telephone), clarifying whether the sequence was concealed until interventions were assigned.
Randomization -- Implementation	Who generated the allocation sequence, who enrolled participants, and who assigned participants to their groups
Blinding (masking)	Whether or not participants, those administering the interventions, and those assessing the outcomes were blinded to group assignment. When relevant, how the success of blinding was evaluated
Statistical methods	Statistical methods used to compare groups for primary outcome(s); Methods for additional analyses, such as subgroup analyses and adjusted analyses

Table 7.15 (Continued)

Topic	Description
RESULTS	Flow of participants through each stage (a diagram is strongly recommended).
Participant flow	Specifically, for each group report the numbers of participants randomly assigned, receiving intended treatment, completing the study protocol, and analyzed for the primary outcome. Describe protocol deviations from study as planned, together with reasons
Recruitment	Dates defining the periods of recruitment and follow-up
Baseline data	Baseline demographic and clinical characteristics of each group
Numbers analyzed	Number of participants (denominator) in each group included in each analysis and whether the analysis was by "intention-to-treat". State the results in absolute numbers when feasible (*e.g.*, 10/20, not 50%)
Outcomes and estimation	For each primary and secondary outcome, a summary of results for each group, and the estimated effect size and its precision (*e.g.*, 95% confidence interval)
Ancillary analyses	Address multiplicity by reporting any other analyses performed, including subgroup analyses and adjusted analyses, indicating those pre-specified and those exploratory
Adverse events	All important adverse events or side effects in each intervention group
DISCUSSION	Interpretation of the results, taking into account study hypotheses, sources of
Interpretation	potential bias or imprecision and the dangers associated with multiplicity of analyses and outcomes
Generalizability	Generalizability (external validity) of the trial findings
Overall evidence	General interpretation of the results in the context of current evidence

APPLYING TRIAL RESULTS TO PATIENT CARE

Lastly, it is necessary to assess the extent to which trial findings (a) provide a valid basis for making generalizations to settings and groups beyond the trial, and (b) apply to individuals. The first issue refers to the generalizability (external validity) of randomized trials, which is frequently low (see Table 7.2 for reasons and for possible solutions besides observational studies, which protect the integrity of the context of service delivery). Reports of randomized trials are expected to include the information needed to help assess generalizability (Table 7.15). Secondly, checklists of issues and questions are also available [14 26] to help assess the applicability of trial results to actual individuals other than the study participants. For example, Dans *et al.* [14] identify 'biologic issues (which help us decide if the treatment can work), socioeconomic issues (which help us decide if the treatment will work) and epidemiologic issues (which help us decide how efficient the treatment will be'. However, evidence of applicability may still require observational studies [12].

REFERENCES

[1]   Hague W, Gebski V, Keech A. Recruitment to randomised studies. *Med. J. Aust.* 2003;178:579-81

[2]   Penston J. Large-scale randomised trials - a misguided approach to clinical research. *Med. Hypotheses* 2005;64:651-7.

[3]   Black N. Why we need observational studies to evaluate the effectiveness of health care. *BMJ* 1996;312:1215-8.

[4]   Sackett D, Rosenberg WC, Muir Gray J, Haynes RB, Richardson WS. Evidence based medicine: what it is and what it isn't. *BMJ* 1996;312:71-2.

[5]   Concato J, Shah N, Horowitz R. Randomised controlled trials, observational studies, and the hierarchy of research designs. *N. Eng. J. Med.* 2000;342:1887-92.

[6]   Benson K, Hartz A. A comparision of observational studies and randomised controlled trials. *N. Eng. J. Med.* 2000;342:1878-86.

[7]   Pocock S, Elbourne D. Randomized trials or observational tribulations? *N. Eng. J. Med.* 2000;342:1907-9.

[8]   Miettinen O, Yankelevitz D, Henschke C. Evaluation of screening for a cancer: annotated catechism of the gold standard creed. *J. Eval. Clin. Pract.* 2003;9:145-50.

[9]   Freemantle N. Medicalisation, limits to medicine, or never enough money to go around? *BMJ* 2002;324:864-5.

[10]   Tan S-B, Dear K, Bruzzi P, Machin D. Towards a strategy for randomised clinical trials in rare cancers: an example in childhood S-PNET. *BMJ* 1995;311:1621-5.

[11]   Devereaux P, Bhandari M, Clarke M, Montori V, Cook D, Yusuf S, et al. Need for expertise based randomised controlled trials. *BMJ* 2005;330:88-91.

[12]   Mant D. Can randomised trials inform clinical decisions about individual patients? *Lancet* 1999;353:743-6.

[13]   Kravitz R, Duan N, Braslow J. Evidence-based medicine, heterogeneity of treatment effects, and the trouble with averages. *Milbank Quarterly* 2004;82:661-87.

[14]   Dans A, Dans L, Guyatt G, Richardson S. How to decide on the applicability of clinical trial results to your patient. *JAMA* 1998;279:545-9.

[15]   De Angelis C, Draxen J, Frizelle F, Haug C, Hocy J, Horton R, et al. Is this clinical trial fully registered? A statement from the International Committee of Medical Journal Editors. *Lancet* 2005;365(9464):1827.

[16]   Roland M, Torgerson D. Understanding controlled trials: What are pragmatic trials? *BMJ* 1998;316:285.

[17]   Beller E, Gebski V, Keech A. Randomisation in clinical trials. *Med. J. Aust* .2002;177:565-7.

[18]   Wennberg J, Barry M, Fowler F, Mulley A. Outcomes research, PORTs, and health care reform. *Ann. NY Acad. Sciences* 1993;703:52-62.

[19]   Friedman L, Furberg C, DeMets. *Fundamentals of Clinical trials.* 3rd Edition. New York: Springer, 1998.

[20]   Montori VM, Permanyer-Miralda G, Ferreira-Gonzalez I, Busse JW, Pacheco-Huergo V, Bryant D, et al. Validity of composite end points in clinical trials. *BMJ* 2005;330:594-6.

[21]   O'Connell R, Gebski V, Keech AC. Making sense of trial results: outcomes and estimation. *Med J Aust* 2004;180:128-30.

[22]   Piantadosi S. *Clinical Trials. A Methodologic Perspective.* New York: John Wiley and Sons, Inc, 1997.

[23] Moher D, Schulz K, Altman D, Group ftC. The CONSORT statement: revised recommendations for improving the quality of reports of parallel-group randomized trials. *JAMA* 2001;285:1897-91.

[24] Campbell M, Elbourne D, Altman D, Group ftC. The CONSORT statement : extension to cluster randomized trials. *BMJ* 2004;328:702-8.

[25] Plint A, Moher D, Morrison A, Schulz K, Altman D, Hill C, et al. Does the CONSORT checklist improve the quality of reports of randomised controlled trials? A systematic review. *Med. J. Aust.* 2006;185:263-7.

[26] Seale J, Gebski V, Keech A. Generalising the results of trials to clinical practice. *Med. J. Aust.* 2004;181:558-60.

Chapter 8

DISSEMINATING RESEARCH

OBJECTIVES

By the time you have completed this chapter, you should be able to

1. Describe how to disseminate your research, in particular by publishing it
2. Write clear, concise and effective prose
3. Avoid major problems with your tables and graphs
4. Suggest how to transfer research knowledge to your target audience

PREVIEW

Until we disseminate our research findings, the journey we have taken in support of all similar quests cannot be 'completed'. This chapter focuses on how to disseminate research, emphasizing one particular strategy: publication. The chapter will summarize the practical knowledge and skills needed to plan, write and publish a manuscript. These issues will be discussed mainly with reference to publishing a Journal paper, but many of the same principles apply to other forms of publication such as book chapters. Lastly, this chapter will elaborate on three sets of components of research outputs: prose, tables and graphs, and maps, before suggesting some steps to help translate research findings into practice.

DISSEMINATING RESEARCH FINDINGS

Dissemination involves sharing findings with others, in particular those who may benefit from using the research. It is important to develop a dissemination plan that can effectively communicate key messages to the target audience in its preferred mode. Crosswaite and Curtice [1] identified three models of dissemination:

1. 'Limestone model:' findings seep into the community and gradually influence policy. Dissemination is characterized by a lack of urgency.

2. 'Gadfly model:' the researcher engages in public relations, actively networking to impress on key individuals the importance of the research.
3. 'Insider model:' the researcher is willing to discuss how to implement findings that are made to reflect the concerns of the commissioners of the research.

Such models view research as a one-way, top-down process of communicating research findings to inform health policy and practice. Critics recommend a two-way process [2], even though this can be resource-intensive and create additional barriers such as power-sharing [3]. They argue that all stages of the research, including dissemination, should involve a systematic and collaborative dialogue between researchers and users in order to help bridge the gap between research and practice. In general, this dialogue should begin early; dissemination should not be afterthought. The dialogue should help to produce a mutual understanding of the needs of the researchers and user groups [4]. It can also be expected to facilitate a shared interest in, understanding of, and sense of ownership over the research process and outcomes, increasing the likelihood that findings will be useful and implemented.

Dissemination can take various forms including informal discussions, newsletters, fact sheets, site reports (e.g., for schools), broadcasts in the popular media (e.g. newspapers, radio, television and the internet), reports at conferences and other meetings (in the form of paper presentations and posters), and publications. It is the last of these modes of dissemination – research publications – that we will consider in detail.

GETTING PUBLISHED

The Latin root of the word 'publish,' *publicare*, means 'to make public.' Table 8.1 summarizes the many steps that are needed to get research published in the public domain, although particularly in academic and professional journals. It identifies individual tasks and suggests how best to manage them. It focuses mainly on publishing papers or articles, since this is the most common publication format among researchers [5 6].

Table 8.1. Steps to Take in Publishing Research

Tasks	How to manage the tasks when uncertain
Determine the need to publish	• People publish for many reasons. Most of these people want to add to knowledge and benefit others. However, other reasons are to get and keep an academic job; for satisfaction, recognition or credibility; and because it's fun!
	• Do not publish to make a fortune. Journals do not pay for the articles they publish; and some journals charge authors to ensure open access to the published papers. Publishers pay royalties to book authors but these are a small proportion of the total sales revenue generated from the book
Choose a topic (key research finding)	• Check that the proposed research is 'new,' i.e. it has not been done before, is new to a particular audience, or updates or expands previous work. To check whether something is worth sharing, apply the 'so what?' test. In general, aim to produce actionable messages that meet an identified need

Table 8.1 (Continued)

Steps to take	Guidance on how
Decide on the type of submission	In general, choose the shortest format appropriate to the message: • Letters • Book reviews • Case reports • Other brief reports • Technical reports • Papers (articles): viewpoints (discussion articles), review articles, original articles • Editorials • Books (Monographs): chapter, edited, authored
Identify the target audience	• Consider who will value and benefit from the message. Key audiences for health research include: service recipients, service providers, managers and policy makers
For papers: identify and select an appropriate Journal	• Use referenced works and the electronic database, 'Journal of Citation Reports (JCR),' to reveal potentially appropriate Journals • Scan these Journals and their 'notes for contributors' to see what types of paper they publish. http://mulford.mco.edu/instr/ provides authors' notes for >3,500 journals in the health and life sciences • Use JCR to help assess the quality of different Journals. Citation impact factors report the number of times, by Journal, that papers published in the past two years have been cited in a given year. Some excellent Journals choose not to have impact factors • Balance the quality of the research, and the target audience, against each Journal's impact factor (or whether/where it is indexed), quality of feedback, rejection rate, and efficiency at reviewing submissions and publishing accepted manuscripts • Query the Editor if necessary • Consider also producing reviews for: The Cochrane Collaboration, The Database of Abstracts of Reviews of Effects (DARE), The Evidence for Policy and Practice Information and Coordinating Centre
Decide on authorship	• Consider including credible authors (who bring research experience, a track record in publishing and high status in the field). They may increase the probability of getting published, even though most journals aim to blind reviewers to the identify of the author(s) • Avoid misunderstandings and ill-will by agreeing on issues relating to the research and authorship (e.g. the division of responsibilities; rights to authorship; authorship order) at the earliest time that is realistic • Read the International Committee of Medical Journal Editors': Uniform Requirements for Manuscripts Submitted to Biomedical Journals: Writing and Editing for Biomedical Publication: http://www.icmje.org/ • This document requires that authors meet three conditions: 1. Substantial contributions to conception and design, or acquisition of data, or analysis and interpretation of data; 2. Drafting the article or revising it critically for important intellectual content; and 3. Final approval of the version to be published And so can 'take public responsibility for appropriate portions of the content.' Participation solely through 'acquisition of funding, collection of data, or general supervision of the research group … does not justify authorship' (see URL above)

Table 8.1 (Continued)

Steps to take	Guidance on how
Structure the paper	The basic structure of original research papers [7] is: • Title: The two types are *indicative* (what the paper covers) and *informative* (the key message of the research, in brief). • Abstract: Summarize the format below. Structured abstracts facilitate this • Introduction: Include the background and a question or problem statement defining the study rationale, aims and any hypotheses • Methods: Describe how the research question was answered, noting the study design, participant attributes, any interventions, data collection methods, and data analysis methods • Results: Describe the findings • Discussion: Summarize and interpret key findings in the light of other, known supporting and conflicting research; discuss strengths and limitations of the study; and consider the implications, e.g. for future research, policy and practice • Conclusion: State the answer to the question posed at the outset In qualitative research, the distinction between results and discussion can blur, but some journals still require a structure that separates them
Begin to write	• Assemble all the materials needed to write the paper; this includes the materials for which permission to use may be required • Select relevant sections e.g. on methods, that can be adapted from any grant application supporting the study • Produce any tables or figures before writing up the results • In general, write the easiest parts first

Revise the paper, including the final manuscript	• Expect to revise the drafts many times
	• Take frequent breaks. Taking time out between drafts allows us to step back and reflect on our progress in crafting the paper
	• Be self-critical and welcome critical feedback from co-authors on early drafts
	• Check that the paper, in accordance with the requirements of the Journal:
	  1. Numbers its pages (with drafts dated or numbered)
	  2. Meets the word limits
	  3. Is formatted appropriately (e.g. font, font size, double spacing)
	  4. Has an accurate and succinct title, plus author details
	  5. Includes an accurate, complete and concise abstract, plus 'key words' for indexing the paper
	  6. Poses a clear and relevant question in the Introduction
	  7. Says everything necessary without being repetitive or long-winded
	  8. Has an appropriate structure, including text headings and subheadings
	  9. Uses accurate, brief, clear – and, if appropriate, punchy prose
	  10. Reports text that agrees with any tables and graphs
	  11. Reaches appropriate and useful conclusions
	  12. Does not omit necessary citations or include unnecessary ones.
	  13. Has had its references checked for content. order and format
	  14. Makes appropriate acknowledgements, e.g. for funding support
	  15. Includes each table or figure on a separate sheet
	• Colleagues who are not co-authors can usefully be asked to read late drafts, as they can bring a detached objectivity

Table 8.1 (Continued)

Steps to take	Guidance on how

Submit the paper for possible publication	• Submit the paper to one journal at a time
	• Send the Editor the full paper (and any copies requested) in the format required by the Journal and using the means specified (e.g. email, post)
	• Include a short, polite covering letter (also called a submission letter)
	• Some Journals require use of their electronic submission systems
	• Include any information that may assist the Editor, for example:
	  1. The type of paper
	  2. Why this Journal was selected
	  3. Assurance that the content of the paper has not been published before and is not being submitted elsewhere
	  4. Any conditions or restrictions that apply on the publication of the paper
	  5. Suggested reviewers
	  6. Full contact details
	• Do not tell the Editor how important the paper is! This should be clear from the paper itself
	• Keep a copy of all material submitted
	• Await an acknowledgement of receipt and, if the paper is sent out to reviewers, the decision of the Editor (usually within three months)

Respond to the Editor's decision	• Look for comments we can learn from and use to improve the paper • Revise the paper, if encouraged to do so, usually within about four weeks and then return it to the journal Editor. Few authors have their papers accepted without revisions, which may be minor or major • Include a letter noting the changes made – or not made for stated reasons. The Editor may seek further reviews on a significantly revised paper • Consider asking for permission to revise a rejected paper in order to meet major objections. It is probably better to revise the paper, submit it elsewhere and log the submission. However, we can appeal a rejection if, on reflection, we believe that the decision is wrong • Once the paper is accepted (although sometimes before), expect to be asked to sign the publisher's copyright form. Meet this request without delay to expedite processing of the paper • Check the copyedited and typeset paper once this is received from the Publisher. Promptly respond to the Publisher's queries, make only minor editorial changes and return the proof to the Publisher • Cite the paper as 'in press.' Make sure that it is published, since errors can happen. Publishers typically provide authors with some free copies of the publication around the time it goes to print

PROSE

Having provided an overview of the publication process, we will now elaborate on individual research components that contribute to the effectiveness and publishability of research outputs. The first of these components is prose that professionally communicates the intended message clearly, concisely, precisely and in a manner engaging readers of the work. Table 8.2 suggests how to produce prose with these attributes, and offers examples of good and poor prose respectively. Numerous style guides are available on how to craft effective prose [8].

Table 8.2. Writing Prose That Works

	Steps to take	Examples of poor prose	Examples of good prose
Accuracy	Use words correctly. Take care with misused word pairs	She was disinterested in going to the clinic	She was uninterested in going to the clinic
	Be gender neutral	A patient should be able to choose the doctor he wants	Patients should be able to choose the doctor they want
	Check spelling, syntax and grammar	Considering the circumstances, the result was pleasing	Considering the circumstances, we are pleased with the result
	Use the correct verb tense	In 2000, Smith has reported …	In 2000, Smith reported …
	Keep sentences and paragraphs short	'After careful consideration of all of the evidence amassed, it is now clear to us that the only valid conclusion is that the doctor was negligent is his failure to disclose to the patients all of the risks of which they could reasonably expect to be fully informed	All the evidence tells us that the doctor was negligent in not telling patients the risks they could reasonably expect to be told
Brevity	Avoid empty phrases	A majority of	Most
		Prior to	Before
		In order to	To
		Through the use of	By
		In the event that	If
		It is clear that	Clearly
		It is possible that the result is	The result may be
		Due to the fact that	Because
		There are many nurses who give	Many nurses give …

Table 8.2 (Continued)

	Steps to take	Examples of poor prose	Examples of good prose
Clarity	Be clear; e.g. avoid obscure language. Exclude jargon unless the audience will understand it	The patient with an exaggerated kyphotic angle from the normal kyphotic curve of her spine	The patient with curvature of her spine (humpback or hunchback)
	Use the active voice where possible	It was decided	We decided
	Use active verbs	Take into consideration	Consider
	Use parentheses sparingly. If what we want to parenthesize is short, consider using commas; if it is long, make it a separate sentence	The rights of the patients (e.g. to have access to their own health records) were specified in the charter	The charter specified the rights of patients, for example to have access to their own health records
	Explain abbreviations before using them	The WHO reported	The World Health Organization (WHO) reported
Concreteness	Write concretely – use 'facts' and specific examples to set the scene	Friendliness is an important attribute	Her smile hinted at her friendliness
Directness	Make points directly and quickly	See the example given in support of brevity	
Engagement	Engage the audience with colorful prose; e.g. paint word pictures with strong metaphors	The doctor was running out of time	The seduction of family practice and illegitimate birth of an expanded role in population health
	Avoid pomposity	It behoves a nurse to take care	A nurse should take care
	Avoid dehumanizing words	Five diabetic cases …	Five people with diabetes …
Formality	Avoid slang and informal phrasings, including clichés, in formal writing	This cystic was	This person with cystic fibrosis was …
	Avoid contractions	He's attending the practice	He is attending the practice

Table 8.3. Effective Tables and Graphs

	Tables	Graphs
Purpose	Visually summarize precise and structured numeric information	Portray numeric trends or relationships, and make comparisons pictorially
Advantages	Show the detailed picture – e.g. by listing or comparing exact numeric values *ACCENT principles of effective tables and graphs:* **Apprehension:** Make patterns readily apprehensible **Clarity:** Ensure that the most important elements or relationships are visually clear **Consistency:** Make the format consistent, internally and with other tables and graphs in the same work **Efficiency:** Present meaningful results as economically and simply as possible **Necessity:** Use the material and format that are needed to best communicate the key message **Truthfulness:** Presents results honestly Adapted from: http://www.math.yorku.ca/SCS/Gallery/	Manage large amounts of data in an efficient and coherent manner Give a quick and forceful sense of patterns More interesting than tables or text
Disadvantages	Less able than graphs to quickly show the big picture and relationships among many variables	Less able than tables to depict the fine picture Time-consuming to produce Technical in form Can be costly to produce

Table 8.3 (Continued)

Tables	Graphs

Tips

- Use the title to convey important information clearly and concisely
- Ensure that the meaning of the table or graph is self-explanatory, but also referred to in the main text with key points highlighted
- Check for any Journal limits (in Notes for Contributors) on numbers of tables or graphs
- Group information logically
- Select appropriate units of measurement and use appropriate intervals (e.g. age ≥ 65 years)
- Use easy-to-read fonts such as Arial, Helvetica and Times Roman
- Avoid abbreviations
- Keep simple, e.g. include no more than three variables
- Compare similar units
- Put close together the numbers to be compared (usually in a column)
- Consider including a row and/or column of contrasts (e.g. column 1 minus column 2)
- Specify the sample size
- Produce no more than nine columns
- Avoid tables containing many empty cells
- Label clearly each column and row.
- Use font weight to distinguish headings from cells entries
- Use label nesting to show relationships: e.g.
- Female patient
  - Male doctor
  - Female doctor
- Report row and column totals
- Align numbers and headings
- Minimize the use of decimal places

Graphs tips:

- Shape the graph to best illustrate the structure of the data, or use the 'golden rectangle' in which the 'aspect ratio' of the width to the height is about 1.3 : 1
- Choose axes limits to reflect the data range, with all areas used
- Use a 'broken y-axis' to preserve a zero base or prevent one or two very large values dominating

- To compare relative (proportional) changes, consider using index numbers or a logarithmic scale on the y axis (equal distances represent equal ratios) and an ordinary arithmetic scale on the x axis. Logarithmic scales cannot show zeroes or negative values
- Avoid 3-dimensional presentations of 2-dimensional data

Table 8.3 (Continued)

Tables	Graphs
• Right justify cell entries • Use footnotes to explain abbreviations, codes and symbols	• Leave discrete points unconnected (unless an interpolation makes sense) • Do not produce pie graphs unless the number of categories is small and sum of individual values is meaningful • Label all axes and use string labels to represent categorical variables • Place labels in (otherwise) unused areas • Use legends only when necessary and order items as they appear in the graph • Avoid the moiré effect by using solid, rather than hatched, fill patterns and by minimizing the space between bars • Try to minimize 'non-data ink', i.e. grids, ticks and frames • Increase clarity by minimizing the use of line styles and symbols

TABLES, GRAPHS AND MAPS

Empirical health research commonly includes tables and figures, such as graphs, in the place of lengthy prose. Table 8.3 describes, evaluates and facilitates the use of tables and graphs in order to help emphasize and communicate the meaning of detailed, numeric results. In turn, maps store abstract geographic representations of selected spatial information. Table 8.4 summarizes effective thematic maps, describing why they are sometimes used, what their production and presentation requires, how they can take different forms, and general tips on producing them.

TRANSLATING RESEARCH INTO PRACTICE

A significant gap exists in health care between what is known and what is done in health care. However, recent years have seen increased interest in moving from research evidence to its implementation in practice. This process of 'knowledge translation' has been conceptualized in various ways. One of these involves moving from awareness through acceptance to adoption [9] and then adherence [10]. In turn, this model has been related to three types of interventions – predisposing, enabling and reinforcing – at different stages of the change process [11]. Table 8.5 summarizes some of the key, practical strategies for meeting requirements of these stages [12, 13].

Table 8.4. Effective Thematic Maps

Thematic maps	Description	Advantages	Disadvantages
Purpose	Show spatial data on a single, specific topic. Record, store and present data in a way that helps people to visualize and conceptualize patterns and processes in space		
Principles	Maps require FAKTS: **F**rame **A**rrow pointing north **K**ey (or legend) **T**itle **S**cale		
Types *Point maps*			
Dot maps	Place dots to represent geographically discrete events of a specific quantity	• Are effective when there are only small contrasts between the mapped phenomenon	• Are visually imprecise • Require a lot of data • Can result in excessive dot coalescence, making distribution patterns difficult to discern

Table 8.4 (Continued)

Thematic maps	Description	Advantages	Disadvantages
Proportional circles maps	Position circles whose area is proportional to the size of the study variable	• Can be combined with dot maps and pie charts	• Can lead people to underestimate the sizes of larger circles and, in particular, larger spheres, relative to smaller ones
Proportional spheres maps	Position spheres whose size is proportional to the size of the study variable	• Can cope with extreme contrasts	
Area-based maps			
Choropleth maps	Shade pre-defined areas in different intensities to represent variability in the mapped data	• Are suited to well-defined groups or classes • Are easy to produce and interpret	• Can falsely suggest abrupt change at area boundaries • Is unable to show variability within areas, necessitating small areas • Can make it difficult to distinguish between class shadings
Isopleth maps	Produce lines that connect, through interpolation, points of equal value on the mapped variable. May also interpolate values between lines	• Are suited to showing gradual change over space in continuous data	• Require a relatively dense scatter of continuous control points
Flow maps	Use lines of varied width (and/or color) to indicate direction and amount of movement in space	• Reduce visual clutter	• Are difficult to produce because computer algorithms are not readily available

Tips
Graytones to indicate intensity, e.g. population density
Hue to show qualitative and intensity differences
Orientation to show flows
Shapes (symbols – points, lines, areas) to show qualitative differences, e.g. a road versus a railway
Texture to show qualitative and intensity differences
Size of point symbols to indicate *magnitude*

Table 8.5. Knowledge Translation

- Publish research to increase its credibility
- Tailor the message and knowledge transfer approach to the target audience
- In general, attempt to use interactive processes (involving direct contact with key representatives of the target audience) rather than passive processes
- Obtain and use budgetary resources to get to know the target audience, including its needs, and to involve its representatives in the research process (action research)
- Share an abstract or full copy of the research report with representatives of the target audience, and spend time with them discussing the findings
- Undertake research relevant to the needs of the target audience, and make this audience aware of what its members can learn from the research
- Develop relationships, and work with intermediaries (e.g. opinion leaders and knowledge brokers, such as journalists) and with researchers similarly engaged in knowledge transfer
- Employ staff with knowledge transfer responsibilities, and invest in the development of knowledge transfer skills among research staff
- Keep abreast of the research literature on knowledge transfer
- Evaluate our own research transfer activities to find out what works for us: assess not just whether decision-makers use our research but how much of it they use and in what ways
- Consider developing and using infrastructure (e.g. websites or newsletters) to support interactive efforts to transfer research knowledge

REFERENCES

[1]   Crosswaite C, Curtice L. Dissemination of Research for Health Promotion: A Literature Review. Edinburgh.: *Research Unit in Health and Behavioural Change*, 1991.

[2]   King L, Hawe P, Wise M. Making dissemination a two-way process. *Health Promot Int* 1998;13:237-44.

[3]   Mason D, Chandler J. Editors introduction to sociology and the policy process—the skills task force. *Sociology* 1999;33:619–38.

[4]   Philip K, Backett-Milburn K, Cunningham-Burley S, Davis JB. Practising what we preach? A practical approach to bringing research, policy and practice together in relation to children and health inequalities. *Health Educ. Res.* 2003;18:568-79.

[5]   Huth E. *How to write and publish papers in the medical sciences*. Philadelphia: ISI Press, 1983.

[6]   Parsell G, Bligh J. AMEE Guide No. 17: Writing for journal publication. *Med. Teacher* 1999;21:457-68.

[7]   Perneger T, Hudelson P. Writing a research article: advice to beginners. *Int. J. Qual. Health Care* 2004;16:191-2.

[8]   Gowers E. *The Complete Plain Words*, 1954.

[9] Davis D, Taylor-Vaisey A. Translating guidelines into practice: A systematic review of theoretic concepts, practical experience, and research evidence in the adoption of clinical practice guidelines. *Can. Med. Assoc. J.* 1997;157:408-16.

[10] Pathman D, Konrad T, Freed G, Freeman V, Koch G. The awareness-to-adherence model of the steps to clinical guideline compliance: the case of pediatric vaccine recommendations. *Med. Care* 1996;34:873-89.

[11] Davis D. The case for knowledge translation: shortening the journey from evidence to effect. *BMJ* 2003;327:33-5.

[12] Lavis J, Ross S, Hurley E. Examining the role of health services research in public policymaking. *Milbank Q* 2002;80:125-54.

[13] Lavis J, Robertson D, Woodside J, McLeod C, Abelson J, Group. KTS. How can research organizations more effectively transfer research knowledge to decision makers? *Milbank Q* 2003;81:221-48.

INDEX